8. 7. 08

D0231722

Language and Clinical Communication

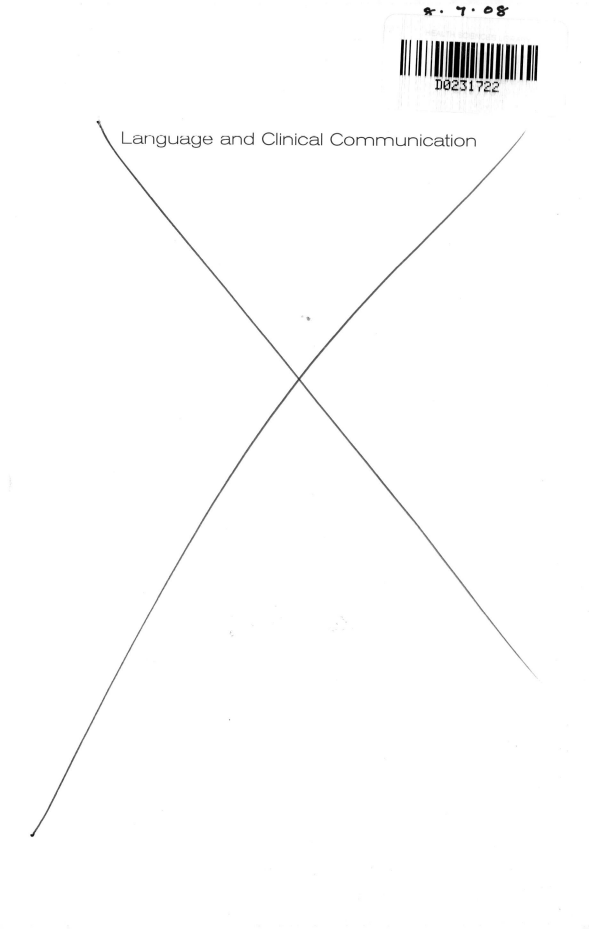

8 . 1 . 68

Language and Clinical Communication

THIS BRIGHT BABYLON

JOHN SKELTON

Director, Interactive Studies Unit
Department of Primary Care and General Practice
University of Birmingham

HM 251
Skelton
H0803638

Radcliffe Publishing
Oxford • New York

Radcliffe Publishing Ltd
18 Marcham Road
Abingdon
Oxon OX14 1AA
United Kingdom

www.radcliffe-oxford.com
Electronic catalogue and worldwide online ordering facility.

© 2008 John Skelton

John Skelton has asserted his right under the Copyright, Designs and Patents Act 1998 to be identified as the author of this work.

All rights reserved. No part of this publication may be reproduced, stored in a retrieval system or transmitted, in any form or by any means, electronic, mechanical, photocopying, recording or otherwise, without the prior permission of the copyright owner.

British Library Cataloguing in Publication Data

A catalogue record for this book is available from the British Library.

ISBN-13: 978 1 84619 125 1

Typeset by Pindar New Zealand (Egan Reid), Auckland, New Zealand
Printed and bound by TJI Digital, Padstow, Cornwall, UK

Contents

Preface

One of my principal professional responsibilities – not to say pleasures – over the last 15 years has been to run the Interactive Studies Unit (ISU) at the University of Birmingham Medical School. All told, we deliver teaching in communication to around 2000 health professionals and students of the health professions each year. Much of what I think I understand about clinical communication has inevitably come, therefore, from the privilege of working alongside colleagues in the core ISU team, and in the wider Department of Primary Care and General Practice of which they are part.

This is a book which I think, and hope, questions more received wisdom than it seeks to confirm. I need therefore to emphasise the strength of the clinical communication tradition, and how much I have gained from it in an understanding of the issues. Everyone who works in this field is aware of a line of enquiry, and beyond that an understanding of the nature of the medical encounter, which began with Balint, perhaps, and has been elaborated, explored and exemplified ever since. It is because of the work of some dozens of influential figures that communication is taken seriously today, and it is their work that makes possible the kind of dialogue with the reader I embark on in this book.

I am also deeply indebted to my wife, Liz, and to Anna and Alice, for their help and support in this and everything.

John Skelton
January 2008

About the author

John Skelton is Director of the Interactive Studies Unit (ISU) at Birmingham University Medical School, where he is Professor of Clinical Communication. He is also Associate Dean for Educational Quality, and Director of the Medical School Education Unit. John is a literature graduate who, before getting involved in medical education, worked as a language teacher, teacher educator and applied linguist in Spain, Oman, Singapore and the UK. He still maintains his interest in education overseas, and has undertaken short consultancies in two dozen countries.

It hung before him this morning, the vast bright Babylon, like some huge iridescent object, a jewel brilliant and hard, in which parts were not to be discriminated nor differences comfortably marked. It twinkled and trembled and melted together, and what seemed all surface one moment seemed all depth the next.

(Lambert Strether reflects on the nature of Paris,
in *The Ambassadors*, by Henry James)

CHAPTER 1

Introduction

> [Teaching involves] hinting, suggesting, urging, coaxing, encouraging, guiding, pointing out, conversing, instructing, informing, narrating, lecturing, demonstrating, exercising, testing, examining, criticizing, correcting, tutoring, drilling and so on – everything, indeed, which does not belie the engagement to impart an understanding. And learning may be looking, listening, overhearing, reading, receiving suggestions, submitting to guidance, committing to memory, asking questions, discussing, experimenting, practising, taking notes, recording, re-expressing and so on – anything which does not belie the engagement to think and to understand.
>
> Michael Oakeshott[1]

Surface, depth and other oppositions

This is a book about clinical communication and clinical education. It is a book, I'm tempted to say, in which problems are posed which are not so very unfamiliar. My point in undertaking it is to elucidate the issues from a different perspective, and in consequence to offer people ways of thinking and reflecting on them which may not have occurred. And I have a further ambition, which is to confirm that what constitutes 'good communication' is so uncertain, context-dependent and subjective that any context-free generalisations we come up with are likely to be banal. From which I think it follows that those of us who are involved in the discipline should embrace a degree of wise subjectivity.

My starting point is with 'surface' and 'depth', with the way what we apparently say is not what we apparently mean, and the way in which the things

1

we do in professional life do and do not mirror the way we are underneath. It is similarly about the extent to which the data that we collect measure and fail to measure what we need to have information about. The book is also partly concerned with other well-established sets of educational oppositions. It draws on notions which are standard in linguistics since Chomsky[2] about the difference between how we 'perform' on particular occasions, and what this says about our underlying 'competence' – and it is about the distinction between 'training' and 'education.'

Rethans *et al.*[3] describe the performance/competence distinction which, although it was originally concerned specifically with language, is often extended to other areas. Thus, they claim, we should differentiate between 'what a doctor actually does in daily practice (performance) and what he or she is capable of doing (competence).' For example, I have what is called 'native-speaker competence' in English, but if I'm tired, or talking too quickly, or inattentive for some reason, I will make mistakes in the actual 'performance.' So this morning as I came to work I got stuck behind a bus: 'boody blus', I muttered. A spoonerism like this is a simple, common type of performance slip, and you can deduce nothing much about my underlying competence in the English language from such things in isolation. *Competence* is what I can do, whereas *performance* is what I actually do on specific occasions.

A word of warning, however. Within medical education the distinction is seldom consistently maintained, and the terms have come to be used in a variety of less theoretically exact ways. Epstein's review article,[4] drawing on an earlier study,[5] says for example:

> [Competence is] the habitual and judicious use of communication, knowledge, technical skills, clinical reasoning, emotions, values, and reflection in daily practice for the benefit of the individuals and communities being served.

'Performance', on the other hand, is 'what [the doctor] does habitually when not observed.' And 'all clinicians may perform at a lower level of competence when they are tired, distracted, or annoyed.' In precise Chomskyean terms, this ought simply to read 'all clinicians perform less well when they are tired, distracted or annoyed.' Strictly, the doctors' level of competence remains the same. Similarly, in the above quotation, the doctor may indeed 'habitually' perform at a similar level, but neither the question of habit nor the lack of observation is integral to the original use of the terms.

I have laboured this point not to make a criticism, but to draw attention to the way in which terms developed within one academic community can get picked up by another, and then develop a life of their own. Thus neither Rethans *et al.* nor Epstein cite Chomsky as a source – Chomsky's own inspiration here, it is generally acknowledged, being the great Swiss linguist, de Saussure.[6] These are aspects of the workings of a 'discourse community', which I discuss in Chapter 3.

At any rate, I shall try to follow Chomsky's usage although, particularly in Chapter 7, I use the word 'performance' in the actor's sense as well.

'Surface' and 'depth' is also a Chomskyean distinction, but I shall use it loosely to distinguish between what we perceive – for example, when we observe communication happening – and what we cannot perceive. The precise meanings of these terms have in any case shifted somewhat over the years within linguistics (and the key phrase 'deep structure' – which has a highly technical meaning – in fact pre-dates Chomsky, as Crystal[7] points out).

The training/education distinction is compactly and lucidly described by Playdon and Goodsman:[8]

> We identify training as a learning process which deals with known outcomes. It is exemplified in the production line and production management, and its central concern is that the same product should be produced identically each time. So it deals in repetitive skills and uniform performances which are expressed as standards or criteria which must be followed exactly. Medicine deals with some areas where uniformity of this kind is desirable – for example, taking blood. But, clearly, these protocols are not the whole of medicine.
>
> For that we must turn to education. Education is a learning process which deals with unknown outcomes, with circumstances which require a complex synthesis of knowledge, skills, and experience to solve problems which are often one-off problems. There are no simple answers to ethically based questions such as 'Should this 3-year-old child have a bone marrow transplant?' Education, on the other hand, refers its questions and actions to principles and values, rather than merely standards and criteria.

Surface and depth, performance and competence, training and education – to which one might add such pairings as rote learning and deep learning, skills and abilities – all of these oppositions catch elements of the most basic of all educational playthings, namely the relationship between appearance and what lies beneath it. And it is the consequences of these issues which are explored in what follows. As a result, I hope, this book will appear as an invitation to think less superficially about what clinical communication is, about what kind of teaching it involves, and about how it can be conceptualised.

I discuss what might be called a form of 'reductionism', but this is a word I dislike. Largely I am wary of it because it has irredeemably negative connotations and is impossible to use fairly. And in fact the thrust of my overall argument – hence the reference to Henry James's ambiguous jewel in the title – is not that 'reductionism is wrong' in some imprecisely general sense, but that it is very hard to tell when splitting concepts into their component parts is a good idea and when it is not. Actually I would want to argue that the real problem we have in clinical communication is simply that we are insufficiently aware of the difficulty. We may split at the right time, we may do it at the wrong time, but we don't discuss it, and because we don't discuss it, we don't appreciate the implications of our choices. And – this being the point at which I admit exasperation – although we often need to atomise, we should not be seduced into a belief that because the result looks in some vague way more scientific it is actually better, or offers more precision, or that the whole is precisely the sum of the splintered parts we are left with. We should, in other words, not ask the sets of often clumsy behavioural categories our energetic atomisation leaves us with to carry more weight than they will bear.

Partly too 'reductionism' is a word that is often misused, as Pinker[9] points out. And, as it is, there are quite enough technical terms in the relevant area of education which are floating around with no very secure moorings. So I have tried to avoid it – sometimes, you may feel, at the expense of unnecessary circumlocution.

A basic argument

My argument is, I think, fairly straightforward.

The search for a set of skills which can be identified and taught as 'good clinical communication' has been of considerable value in persuading decision makers at medical schools and other bodies that communication matters. These days, very large numbers of medical schools use what are essentially skills-based models, such as the extraordinarily thorough Calgary–Cambridge[10] approach. However, I believe that the emphasis on 'communication' as simply a set of skills, such as eye contact, open questions and so on, has badly skewed the development of the discipline. The teaching of 'communication *skills*' in fact strikes me as a very small part of what I do, not a very difficult part for the majority of students, and – whisper it – one which is often pretty dull.

Yet there is, in the literature and in the persistent use of the label itself, an emphasis on communication as a set of surface skills. The reasons for this are clear enough. First, 'skills' are generally (although not invariably) conceived of as elements of perceptible behaviour. We can see eye contact, we can hear open questions, and we know – or think we know – how such skills can be defined. And, being perceptible, these skills are amenable to empirical research.

Secondly – a point not usually made, but not contentious – part of the definition of communication is that it is perceptible. It may not actually be perceived (I may not hear you over the traffic noise), but it is perceptible, in the sense that it is capable of being perceived. It therefore, prima facie, lends itself perfectly to the kind of research paradigms that are familiar in the sciences.

However, the action of communication on the hearer, to put the case at its simplest – and most extreme – is not the same as the action of a drug on a patient. Nor can 'poor communication' be identified with the objective ease of (many) clinical conditions. In the end, good communication fulfils a set of aims which are abstract and not susceptible to simple definitions. It is perverse to ask 'What is "empathy"?' and expect an answer of the kind one gets to the question 'What is "pneumonia"?'

The difficulty is compounded by societal and educational demands for transparency. For example, research ought to tell us what is the case. Curriculum design ought to make clear selections from research about what should be taught. Students should be clear that the transparently stated curriculum outcomes are what will be tested. So for all these elements of the educational endeavour, we talk of perceptible behaviours. And this is a very good thing, in many ways. Indeed, we mirror it in classroom practice, talking not of 'empathy' in the abstract, but giving students opportunities to practise it – for example, in a simulation. And if we are ever asked 'What is "empathy"?', we can therefore reply 'Well, you remember when you said "Oh dear", and leaned towards your patient? That was being empathic.' That was *empathy in action* – that was *doing empathy*. And, we might feel with a certain glow of satisfaction, that is exactly what good feedback is like – evidence based.

Put like this, what we have is an inductive ('bottom-up') syllabus in action. The so-called 'traditional' syllabus works deductively (it is 'top down'). It begins with the assertion of grand principles ('The main symptoms of X are . . .') and invites learners to observe them in practice subsequently. The inductive syllabus invites learners to reach their own generalisations from a string of particular examples. 'So', we might say to our student, 'here are not one but a dozen examples of the abstract term "empathy." Now is it clear what empathy is?'

This is an excellent way of proceeding. Abstract terms need to be demonstrated. Within medical education, this kind of approach is entirely consonant with the general principles of problem-based learning. Incidentally, one of the driving forces in this kind of approach, as in a substantial amount of education over the last half century and beyond, has been language teaching. Some of the principles are well elucidated in Julian Dakin's early classic.[11] (Dakin was a precocious talent who died tragically young.) They don't, however, sit very easily with the desire to keep things at the level of absolute transparency, as

I shall argue. Dakin's general approach to teaching and learning is usually described as 'mentalist.' And in that term, which drives a great deal of the learning endeavour into the mind, where it can no longer be perceived, lie the seeds of the problem.

Things, in other words, are not simple. To speak of transparency, to teach and test and research and set goals and all the rest of it as clearly as possible, is to risk impoverishment of the discipline – or, as some might phrase it, to turn a potential for education into an occasion for training, with this latter term carrying all kinds of negative connotations, at worst of unthinking rote learning.

The danger is well illustrated in aspects of the current debate about 'professionalism', which is a contemporary growth area in medical education, and one which overlaps with communication in a number of ways. This is an attempt, at its most basic level, to respond to the problem that there are people capable of passing examinations of clinical knowledge and understanding, and capable of mastering clinical skills, who nevertheless ought not to be doctors. Much of the work from the USA on this topic is directly or indirectly motivated by 'Project Professionalism',[12] and the central debates are well set out in Stern *et al.*[13]

Clearly, 'professionalism' as a concept is abstract. It consists, let us say, of a sense of duty, probity, honesty and a great many other virtues which are hard to define. One strand of the debate therefore is that we should consider not the abstract qualities, but their manifestation as surface behaviour.[14,15] Thus a virtuous doctor will (say) turn up at work on time, and so on. They will demonstrate perceptible behaviour which will 'do virtue', in the same way that the student described above was doing empathy. Such behaviour is perceptible, and this perceptibility makes it easier to handle and discuss than the abstract concepts that specific behaviours exemplify. The point is picked up and echoed by van de Camp *et al.*:[16]

> ... students do not identify themselves with elements of professionalism such as 'duty' and 'honour', ... they define professionalism in practical terms such as 'not causing physical harm to patients.' Hence, by framing professionalism in terms of behaviour, we come much closer to a context-bound, realistic framework for understanding professional behaviour.

Neither students nor faculty, it is argued, appear to understand such words particularly clearly in the abstract. Ginsburg *et al.*[17] here quote Phelan *et al.*:[18]

> [Faculty] have been found to have 'difficulty in identifying problems, an inability to verify problems, and fear of litigation' that inhibit their reporting of behavioural problems.

This outcome arises, in part, from the fact that educators and researchers have traditionally focused on this problem from an abstract perspective. The definitions and subcategories of the broader concept of professionalism describe the idealized person, the 'consummate professional', with no room for mistakes. With this theoretical basis, if someone tells a lie, even for a 'good' reason, he or she could be suddenly labelled 'dishonest', and therefore 'unprofessional.' The only thing left for the evaluator to decide, then, is how unprofessional the individual is. This top-down focus on professionalism as an abstraction rather than a bottom-up focus on professionalism as a set of actions in context, therefore, is flawed.

If we are to assess fairly, we must share an understanding of what we are assessing, and that must mean that we know what we mean when we say that an individual is 'dishonest.' 'Duty' is like 'empathy' – a vaguer word, and a concept that is harder to grasp than 'pneumonia.' However, it hardly follows that we ought not to use abstract terms when we teach, or explore what they mean. The problem (I don't claim that the writers I mention above fall victim to this when they teach) is that one might end up with nothing but the set of examples – with a completely flat, surface structure in which 'duty' is just a list of things to do.

This debate is as old as the hills, or at any rate as old as the Socratic dialogues. Socrates' methodology as a teacher – or rather, this methodology as it is reported by Plato, who was one of his pupils and who wrote the dialogues – was often to begin with just such an abstract term and, by holding it up to the light through questioning, to reveal how poorly we understand it. Here he is in the *Meno*,[19] a dialogue which is, incidentally, one of the cornerstones of western education (a point I pick up in the second book of this series). Socrates has just asked Meno, one of his pupils, what 'being good' is:

> Meno: Well, it's not very difficult, Socrates. If you want to know what being good is *for a man* – well, that's easy. Here's what being a good man is: having what it takes to handle your city's affairs, and, in doing so, to help out your friends and hurt your enemies (while making sure they don't do the same to you). Or, if you want me to explain what being a *good woman* is, no problem: she's got to be good at looking after the home, be thrifty with household goods and always obey her man . . .

And he moves on to how other types of person can be good. Very little of this looks like 'being good' these days, and the passage is a reminder of how our sense of 'goodness' changes over time and place. Socrates responds with a certain amount of lugubrious irony:

> Socrates: Well, what an amazing stroke of luck! There I was, looking for just one sort of 'being good' and it turns out you've brought along a whole swarm of the things . . .

Then, prompted by the word 'swarm', he begins to talk about how there are 'lots of different kinds of bees' yet, clearly, all bees share something, do they not? And he concludes that individual examples of 'goodness' must have 'something that makes them all cases of being good.'

This is the crux of the matter. We may not be able to define 'goodness', or 'professionalism', or any such abstract quality, but it is – they are – more than a set of cases. If we ignore this fact we will encounter problems. In the assessment of professionalism, say, the isolation of behaviours which are assessed would result in students performing them for cynical rather than for virtuous reasons. For communication, doctors could pretend to care by communicating according to a set of rules, and so on. (The question of whether this would actually work is one I shall take up later.)

A standard theological argument for the existence of arbitrary evil is that, if good behaviour were always rewarded and wicked behaviour were always punished, then we would be cynically virtuous, and would not live in a moral universe. I don't mean this suddenly very profound comparison entirely frivolously. If we test professionalism purely by testing behaviour, we remove professionalism from the test. And if we consider communication as the vehicle through which the clinician represents the person he or she is, then the same is true of communication. After all, by some possible definitions of the term, 'communication' would be the *only* vehicle the clinician has to represent who he or she is, if communication is the label we give to how we reach out from our selves to the world beyond us.

Profound ethical issues are inevitably around the edges of many areas touched upon in this book, but I don't intend to pursue them at any length. For example, the points raised by Ginsburg *et al.* above clearly touch upon the standard ethical debate about whether actions are to be judged by the intentions of the agent or the consequences of the action. For our purposes, we can I hope simply agree that good intentions are part of what we want the good doctor to have.

Another important issue is that phrase 'in context', which Ginsburg *et al.* use. Indeed, they make the point repeatedly that the qualities at issue are context dependent. So it is that we have a set of abstract qualities, like 'empathy' and 'duty', expressed in terms of lists of behaviours which sit like burst balloons at the educational party. (Ginsburg *et al.* cite 'introduced self to patient' and 'acknowledged the agenda from the last visit' as examples of 'humanistic skills.' It isn't a way I could use the word 'humanistic', although I know what is meant.) And at the same time, there is a recognition that context changes what the fulfilment of such qualities would consist of in any case, so that it is not the behaviour but the abstract concept which is constant. Either way it seems we are driven into subjective judgements.

And that is the essence of my argument – surface skills are not enough.

Three preoccupations and a confession

Beyond that, I should say a little more about my personal preoccupations, of which I will name three. The first is this. I come from a humanities background. One of the earliest things I read when I got involved in medical education was the Toronto consensus statement,[20] still widely quoted today, and at that time (the early 1990s) the most important single document in the field of medical communication. Its bullish statement that communication skills 'can be defined with behavioural criteria and can be reliably taught and assessed' struck me as simply bizarre. It had never occurred to me to doubt either proposition – except that I would never have wanted to subscribe to the view that they can be *completely* defined by such criteria. Nor had I ever encountered in the real world a moment so Copernican yet so anachronistic, as if the great astronomer were to step forward today to proclaim his heliocentricity, at a time when all the sensible and busy world would glance around and say, 'Well, yes. Very helpful, thanks for that', and look at their watches in a marked manner.

My slow understanding that within the community of academic medicine such a statement was actually necessary has conditioned my thinking to the point where I have a serious interest in two superficially contradictory things. One is a belief that, if anyone is to challenge some of the shakier assertions of the communication skills industry – as they must surely be challenged when the vagaries of fashion allow – the responsible thing is for it to be a communications specialist rather than a doctor who does the challenging. A doctor may simply be thought of as a flat-earther, a Luddite, someone whose exasperation with communication is evidence of a dead soul – or may be taken seriously and allowed to divest medical education of baby and bathwater alike. A specialist in communication may be seen differently – even, sadly, being taken less seriously. In this sense, I want to sound a note of caution about the value of the discipline to the health professions, and about what I believe research has shown. In the end, and with all the normal caveats, the difference between a good communicator and a good doctor is that even if both can talk the good talk, it's the latter who makes you better.

At the same time, I think the label of 'communication skills' is a straitjacket.

It is hopelessly constricting, and confines the discipline to an educational backwater. I have a desire to show how far an understanding of communication can take us as educators.

So in a sense I regard the true worth of communication as both overstated and understated in contemporary educational dialogue. Of course, I would argue, the contradiction is illusory. The point is that although communication *skills* matter less than is often perceived, communication in a wider sense matters more.

Back to my preoccupations. The second one is this. My interest in the study of clinical communication is primarily educational. My research aims are to identify things about the nature of clinical communication which help students of the health professions and qualified health professionals to understand communication better, and as a result to do their job better – of course for the good of patients, but also because the satisfaction of being a good professional is a great vehicle for happiness. I believe, too, that learning in this area presupposes understanding, that this in turn presupposes an ability to reflect, and that an ability to reflect presupposes an ability to articulate ideas.

From this, thirdly, it follows that I do not believe teaching necessarily consists of telling people what is the right thing to do. At its most exciting, teaching involves an enrichment of understanding, with a view to helping learners to develop their own ideas, and – in the case of clinical communication – by extension improving their own skills and deploying them effectively. Education is, in the end, about helping people to think. Hence the quotation from Oakeshott with which I preface this chapter. Oakeshott is generally regarded as a conservatively minded educationalist (whatever that means, I find myself grumbling), and I imagine myself as not being so – but the 'engagement to think and to understand' is what good learning, responsible learning, involves. Or, to put it another way, what matters most to me is education, not training.

In this book I therefore try to address in detail what I think of as the problems in the existing research base, but the reader who is looking for an alternative set of rules for 'effective communication' will be disappointed. There are general tendencies, of course, and these must be taught, but they are not profound and not unexpected. In other words, in response to the challenge 'Well, do you have any better evidence to put before us than what we already know?', I would respond, no doubt irritatingly, that it all depends what you mean by evidence, but the short answer is no. My concern in fact is not so much with the quality of the best evidence, but with the amount of faith we invest in it. And I am concerned, too, about the extent to which we believe our task is done when we have taught all the things that the evidence apparently permits.

On the other hand, if the reader finds nothing that offers him or her a way of reflecting more profoundly on communication, then I in turn will be disappointed. I talk at some length (Chapter 6) about the problems faced by doctors I have worked with. The point of these case histories is to try to elaborate ways in which the surface and the depth of communication differ, to consider how one might seek to address these areas, and to invite the reader directly to question what the limits of the word 'communication' ought to be, or what the task of 'teaching communication' ought to include and exclude.

What are the limits of communication? It is such a pervasive feature of life – we communicate with words, with our hands, with everything from sighs to road signs – that it can be an extraordinarily voracious beast, quite capable of swallowing whole disciplines. We should be very aware of this. It does so in one of two ways. The first of these is to say that the effect of communication is indefinitely large, from which it follows that misuses of language, for instance, have incalculably grave consequences. Most human disasters can probably be repackaged as 'communication problems' if one stretches the term far enough.

Secondly, there is a sense – familiar to students of semiotics – in which everything is a 'sign', everything has the potential to communicate. This is true, of course – the hem coming unstuck on the nurse's uniform, the unmended fence that surrounds the hospital car park, the untidily gathered pieces of paper on the receptionist's desk, and the two young doctors gossiping in the corridor all signify, and therefore communicate, certain things. One of the ways forward for the discipline is to expand into an understanding of the importance of these areas, I believe, but not usefully under the name 'communication skills.' Somewhere one must set limits.

So, at one end of the scale, 'communication' may be interpreted very conservatively. 'Clinical communication' we may declare just *is* nothing more than the set of skills we have been hammering away at over the years. However, I want to go a little way towards the opposite end of the scale (where the world consists only of communication acts), to go beneath the words on the page, or the words that get spoken. The reader may feel that I go too far, or not far enough – that I encroach too much or too little on the territory of other types of expert.

A confession is in order here. I try to make my arguments in a reasoned manner, but the fact is that I find some of the studies which have been done over the last 30 years slightly absurd. In particular, ploddingly serious proof-of-concept studies which demonstrate that it is possible to change someone's observed communication behaviour as a result of training in communication seem to me – and it's a point I have made before[21] – as futile as proof-of-concept studies which demonstrate that training in swimming improves swimming. (My particular problem with this – don't get me started – is the way that column inches in leading journals get filled with earnest attempts to display the elegance of the research design, and leave little room for details of how the teaching was actually conducted, which would be genuinely helpful.)

I have tried in consequence to draw together the strands from my own background, and from related areas. I have also attempted to restrict myself to fairly straightforward arguments, and not to explore the ramifications of the issues I discuss beyond my immediate concern.

In particular, though, my education is literary first of all, and to be educated in literature is to find it making sense of one's professional as well as one's personal life. I have tried to reflect this, and as a result (I suspect rather disingenuously) echo the ambivalence I feel about the way in which many courses in 'Medical Humanities' turn out to be studies of all-the-bits-with-doctors-in from modern classics. I don't have personal experience of literature working like this, of it not being transferable beyond its original setting. Few doctors are regicides like Macbeth, but many do unethical things in pursuit of ambition – whereas the professional significance of the actual doctor in the Scottish play is fairly slight.

Underpinning much of my thinking in this area, in fact, is what I shall call the 'Hamlet question.' (For the literary pedant, I reference the standard Wells and Taylor edition,[22] but reinstate the fuller version of this speech which appeared in the Second Quarto, and which Wells and Taylor give as an 'additional passage.') Hamlet's mother, Gertrude, it will be recalled, has married her dead husband's brother in what Hamlet sees as a lust-driven marriage. He pleads with her to change her ways:

> *Hamlet:*   Good night – but go not to mine uncle's bed.
> Assume a virtue if you have it not.
> That monster custom, who all sense doth eat,
> Of habits devilish, is angel yet in this:
> That to the use of actions fair and good
> He likewise gives a frock or livery
> That aptly is put on. Refrain tonight
> And that shall lend a kind of easiness
> To the next abstinence, the next more easy –
> For use almost can change the stamp of nature . . .

> (III.iv.151ff, plus Q2 additions)

If his mother resists the temptation to continue the sexual liaison with Claudius which Hamlet finds so repulsive, if she modifies her behaviour step by step, so the desire itself will diminish, and her attitude to her new husband will change.

She will no longer wish to pursue an incestuous relationship with a fratricide. This – a kind of Renaissance 'one day at a time' approach – mirrors some aspects of modern views on the handling of addiction problems.

The question for any educator is how far one believes that getting someone into the habit of behaving in a particular way will alter their attitude. Can 'use' 'change the stamp of nature'? For example, if we train medical students to talk courteously to patients, will this make them want to talk courteously to patients? Or would you prefer to say that it was better to get students to reflect on the point of such courtesy, and offer them ways to do it? The former way of approaching things we might want to label, as I have done, 'training', and the latter we might want to label 'education.' My theoretical preference is for the latter, but like most people I do a bit of both, really. However, the reader might like to bear the Hamlet question in mind as we go along.

Finally, I have drawn on the tradition of linguistics to a substantial extent. To the clinician reading this, I would stress that I am not aware of saying anything remarkably original or controversial when it comes to the nature of language.

References

Note: Throughout this book, I have given references to works from fields such as literature and philosophy with regard to ease of availability rather than necessarily referencing standard, or canonical editions. And where there is a significant time lapse between the publication date of the volume I cite and the time at which the original work first appeared – Shakespeare being an obvious example – I give the latter date as well. I have also, for texts legitimately available online, given a number of web references for ease of access. The reader should be aware, however, that this may mean that the edition cited in print form differs from that cited electronically. Plato's *Meno*, for instance, is quoted in print form in the recent Beresford translation, but the online reference is to the more familiar Jowett translation.

1 Oakeshott M. Education: the engagement and its frustrations. In: Dearden RF, Hirst PH, Peters RS, editors. *Education and the Development of Reason.* London: Routledge and Kegan Paul; 1975.
2 Chomsky N. *Aspects of the Theory of Syntax.* Cambridge, MA: MIT Press; 1965.
3 Rethans J-J, Sturmans F, Drop R *et al.* Does competence of general practitioners predict their performance? Comparison between examination setting and actual practice. *BMJ.* 1991; **303:** 1377–80.
4 Epstein RM. Assessment in medical education. *NEJM.* 2007; **356:** 387–96.
5 Epstein RM, Hundert EM. Defining and assessing professional competence. *JAMA.* 2002; **287:** 226–35.

6 Saussure F de (Baskin W, trans.). *Course in General Linguistics.* London: Fontana; 1974. (First published in 1922 as *Cours de Linguistique Générale.* Bally C and Sechehaye A, editors, and reproduced in de Mauro T, Edition Critique. Paris: Payot; 1972.)

7 Crystal D. *A Dictionary of Linguistics and Phonetics* (4e). Oxford: Blackwell; 1997.

8 Playdon Z-J, Goodsman D. Education or training: medicine's learning agenda. *BMJ.* 1997; **314:** 983.

9 Pinker S. *The Blank Slate: the modern denial of human nature.* Harmondsworth: Penguin; 2002.

10 Kurtz S, Silverman J, Draper J. *Teaching and Learning Communication Skills in Medicine.* Oxford: Radcliffe Medical Press; 1998.

11 Dakin J. *The Language Laboratory and Language Learning.* London: Longman; 1973.

12 American Board of Internal Medicine. *Project Professionalism;* www.abim.org/pdf/profess.pdf (accessed 2 April 2007).

13 Stern D, editor. *Measuring Medical Professionalism.* Oxford: Oxford University Press; 2006.

14 Stern DT, Frohna AZ, Gruppen LD. The prediction of professional behaviour. *Med Educ.* 2005; **39:** 75–82.

15 Ginsburg S, Regehr G, Stern D *et al.* The anatomy of the professional lapse: bridging the gap between traditional frameworks and students' perceptions. *Acad Med.* 2002; **77:** 516–22.

16 van de Camp K, Vernooij-Dassen M, Grol R *et al.* Professionalism in general practice: development of an instrument to assess professional behaviour in general practitioner trainees. *Med Educ.* 2006; **40:** 43–50.

17 Ginsburg S, Regehr G, Hatala R *et al.* Context, conflict and resolution: a new conceptual framework for evaluating professionalism. *Acad Med.* 2000; **75 (Suppl. 10):** S6–11.

18 Phelan S, Obenshain S, Galey WR. Evaluation of the non-cognitive professional traits of medical students. *Acad Med.* 1993; **68:** 799–803.

19 Plato (written *c.* 380 BC, Beresford A, trans.). *Meno.* Harmondsworth: Penguin; 2005; http://classics.mit.edu/Plato/meno.html (accessed 23 October 2007).

20 Simpson M, Buckman R, Stewart M *et al.* Doctor–patient communication: the Toronto consensus statement. *BMJ.* 1991; **303:** 1385–7.

21 Skelton JR. Everything you were afraid to ask about communication skills. *Br J Gen Pract.* 2005; **55:** 40–46.

22 Wells S, Taylor G, editors. *The Oxford Shakespeare: the complete works* (2e). Oxford: Oxford University Press; 2005.

CHAPTER 2

The ambiguous inheritance

This is our land. We have our inheritance.

(TS Eliot, Ash Wednesday[1])

Three kinds of audience

The case for communication skills – for teaching, for research, for use with patients – is made routinely these days. Sometimes piously, sometimes cynically, sometimes with a passion real or ersatz, sometimes with a sense of ethical imperative, and sometimes from a less noble sense that that's what one does, because that's how the pendulum is swinging. However, the case may at times seem so often to be made that the issues have lost any power to resonate, and are subscribed to almost from force of habit.

Not by everyone, of course – and one of the difficulties with the present situation is the chasm between those who teach clinical communication, or reflect on it in their practice because it would never cross their mind not to – and, well, everyone else. The former, you would probably agree, are people like us. The latter are strange and irritating beings crouched on the other side of the fence. Some of them indeed, we might say, are dinosaurs, mere mechanics of the body, who grumble in an antediluvian manner that no one ever died from rudeness.

It is the aim of this book, as I say, to look critically and I hope vigorously at the discipline – to reflect on its predilections and problems, and to suggest some ways forward. And to some extent to do so against the backdrop of two simultaneous needs, which may even be contradictory. First, there is the need to reinvigorate and extend the debate about what we mean by 'good clinical communication', and how we know that it is a good idea. Yet, secondly, there is a need to hammer home the central lines of argument to the unconverted, as nearly as possible in a language understood behind the dark, forbidding walls of Jurassic Park. The first requires subtlety. The second does, too, but of a different kind.

So here, then, is the case for research and teaching in clinical communication skills as it is usually made. And, as every case presupposes an audience, we may postulate a series of possibilities here – three versions of the educationally unsophisticated, so not at all like you and I. They share a degree of naivety; they are not the kind of person who would articulate the issues easily.

We might therefore first think in journalistic terms, and have a mental image of someone – a lay person, perhaps, or a patient, as we all are, but not someone with profound experience of the health professions. Someone who has always been well and is at an age where they need not consider too closely the possibility of becoming ill. Someone, that is, who would respond to the sort of journalistic accounts in Table 2.1, taken from a BBC report on an initiative postulated by the (now defunct) NHS University.[2] This is a world where understanding is couched in such pre-theoretical terms as 'gaffes', 'outbursts' and 'bedside manner', where poor communication is explicitly lack of niceness.

Table 2.1 'Clinical Communication' and the media: on being nice

---

Doctors to get lessons on being nice

NHS staff are to receive lessons on how to be nice to patients, under plans being drawn up by the Department of Health.

A training programme to improve the communication skills of newly qualified doctors and nurses is to be established later this year.

Courses for all other NHS staff are expected to be up and running by the middle of next year.

The programme, which will be run by psychologists, will aim to ensure that staff are more sensitive to patients and avoid making gaffes or outbursts . . .

. . . A Department of Health spokeswoman said, 'We want all staff in the NHS to be given training with a patient-centred focus.'

Friday 26 April 2002

Niceness, communication, patient-centredness. The reductive power of the banal word. It isn't the fault of those who planned the programme, or those who were interviewed, that it has come out like this. It makes the point, I suppose, to the first of our putative audiences – that someone out there thinks that doctors should care, and show that they care. And that if they don't, or don't know how to, they should be told. However, this kind of formulation is the soft underbelly of the field. It is, frankly, easy to make communication – communication as a substantive entity – sound vacuous, a label for some vague empathy or other, a version of caring and sharing lifted from the TV confessional, and its moral equivalent. Not, in other words, something that the serious doctor ought to be concerned with, let alone actively engaged in.

This is true even when the research is there in the background, hovering just off-stage, as in this other piece of journalism (*see* Table 2.2).[3]

Table 2.2 'Clinical Communication' and the media: presenting the professional's view

---

Good bedside manners make a difference

With healthcare employers increasingly measuring patient satisfaction levels and rewarding their employees for providing high-quality customer service, health professionals are realizing a good bedside manner is more important than ever. Good bedside manners not only improve interactions with patients, but also advance health professionals' careers . . .

. . . Physicians who communicate well are less likely to be sued for malpractice than poor communicators, says Dr Greg Schneider, assistant professor of family practice and community medicine at UT Southwestern Medical School at Dallas. 'There is a clear association between rapport with patients and incidence of lawsuits.' . . . In addition, Schneider has observed situations where intuitive physicians who have the ability to connect with patients thrive in a group medical practice, while less personable physicians flounder . . .

. . . At Children's Memorial Hospital in Chicago, employees' performance appraisals include an evaluation of soft skills like respect, courtesy, listening and anticipating patients' needs . . .

. . . 'I think there has been a much stronger emphasis on the service aspect of the whole healthcare experience', says Maureen Mahoney, a nurse who is the corporate manager for service excellence at Children's Memorial Hospital. The best way for health workers to learn good bedside manners is by example . . . 'Our leaders need to be good role models for what good bedside manner looks like. You don't necessarily learn some of this in school, but it really makes a difference for patients and families.'

Opinions differ on whether bedside manner can be taught. 'I think [it] can be taught, to an extent, but it does depend a little bit on the raw material', Schneider says. 'I think, ultimately, if you can get someone to appreciate the importance of compassion and coming to an understanding of a patient, they will be able to develop bedside manner. You can teach them some skills in terms of ways to say things and ways to approach difficult topics.' For example, physicians need to be reminded to eliminate medical jargon and check to make sure patients understand what they're being told . . .

. . . The bottom line is that health professionals with good bedside manners may be happier in their jobs, experts say. Mahoney . . . says her most memorable experiences occurred during her days as a bedside nurse. 'You really have an ability to impact on patients' and families' experiences with your organization', she says. 'You can help them heal. Sometimes you feel you don't have the time to sit and have conversations, but you can do little things. You can touch a child's hand, make eye contact or acknowledge their emotions in 30 seconds.'

The appeal to the intuitive, the personable, and the tugging at the heartstrings of the closing image all swamp the other parts of the message – the issue of teachability, of lawsuits, of personal development and personal happiness, even the supposed use of 'jargon' and the checking of understanding. All of these things are discussed in the research, the latter two being items which commonly appear in checklists of good communication, but – through no fault of the interviewees – they vanish beneath a well-meaning, amorphous compassion, a journalist's confection and a reduction to mush of something of value.

Well then, we ought to be tough about what we mean, and present it with backbone, vigour, precision. Evidence, that's the word. Evidence not cheapened by the press. This surely is what we rest our case on. Isn't it? Evidence the whole thing works.

And here is our second audience. Instead of the patient whose interest halts long enough over the website article to note it and drift on, we might now think of doctors of a previous generation, who sensed in their own practice the need for something beyond their clinical skills, who observed in themselves or others that patients sometimes prosper and sometimes do not, who perceived that the whole venture of medicine was rendered easier, more honourable, more effective by holistic care. And who a generation or two ago could only mutter to themselves or colleagues: 'It's a good thing, holistic care – whatever that means, precisely.'

These doctors could, for example, have been training others. They might have found themselves with a young colleague who was somehow less than adequate, although sound enough clinically. Someone who attracted general expressions of disquiet from patients. 'He's a bit brusque', the trainer might have ruminated vaguely. 'A bit high-handed, or a bit shy, a bit reserved.' . . . And other than saying 'Be less brusque', perhaps this senior doctor will have had no means of helping the junior colleague. Lacking the words with which to describe the ill-defined holism they appreciated, they could perhaps have pointed at themselves, but with the uncomfortable feeling that, however valuable the apprenticeship model, 'Watch how I do it' was in the end not in itself a complete training. And then communication skills research came along to help them, to give their thoughts words, their feelings substance, and their consultations structure.

Seen in this context, the plight of the trainer before research, the plight of the discipline of communication – of good communication seen as a part of holistic care – is not unlike the difficulty faced in the first part of the twentieth-century psychology before the advent of Skinner's version of behaviourism. Skinner's role in a kind of muscular purging of consciousness is well understood. His cold passion for replacing the amorphous 'mind' with the precise mechanisms of stimulus and response, his fierce reduction of the human condition to behaviour because it is behaviour that is measurable (it's on the surface, it's perceptible – it's science), played an important part in giving psychology its modern identity, and a place at the contemporary academic table. Behaviour is what a scientist may look at – all the rest is speculation. And this argument, although now old and well worn, is something I shall have to return to at length.

Here, we might tell our second audience, if they are with us still in contemporary life, here is the gift of communication skills research to modern medicine. It offers a vocabulary for things that happen in the consultation, for things that can be measured, evaluated and brought within the scientific scheme of things. Now the trainer has a way of telling the trainee why he or she is not making contact with the patient. Now it is possible to say 'You need to ask open questions more often.' And beyond that, it is possible to say 'Open questions are a good thing.' And finally, it is possible to say 'We know these things.' Or so it is said.

This brings us to our third audience, helpfully sketched for us in the following quotation, which is part of an attack on modern medical education:[4]

> What good are doctors who empathise, smile and maintain eye contact if they do not know their stuff? How much better to have a brusque expert who can prescribe the right course of action.

That word 'brusque' again. The sentiment is of course impossible to disagree with, and for our purposes the tone of voice is helpfully curmudgeonly.

We are, I think, with this kind of individual, still postulating a naif when it comes to communication skills, but one with both power and a scientific training. Perhaps we might imagine someone like this as a decision maker for some organisation or other that funds research, or a dean of a medical school. Perhaps they are of the old school, or the old school as it was said to be and probably wasn't, a thug and a bully in clinical practice, a believer indeed that poor communication kills no one, and that even if it does, well, what can one do? Good communication isn't teachable, you're either born with it or not, some people can do it, others simply can't – a way of putting it which in education usually means 'I have no idea how to teach this.'

Or perhaps they are not like that at all. Perhaps this is someone who accepts perfectly well that their knowledge of communication is limited, that they cannot reasonably be expected to be expert in everything, but perhaps too they are right in their belief that they have an open mind, that they are open to persuasion, that they love innovation, and wish to foster exciting, novel ideas if at all possible. In fact, it hardly matters. The only way to tackle this kind of person, it seems, to address this kind of argument, is to meet them on the field of science, and say 'Here are some things that we know. And now we can do this.'

Dear Dean, one might say. I would like to come and see you, with a view to dragging our medical school out of the fog and mist of a previous era by showing how you might do better than pay irritable lip service to the concept of communication simply because you know we're supposed to. I have that to say which will make you change your mind. It will take just half an hour of your time.

One kind of evidence

So at this stage let us leave behind our lay audience, reassured by the comfortable message of patient-centred caring, which fits so well with contemporary notions of being heard, of being important, of exchanging views in an atmosphere of mutual respect. And let us also leave behind our doctors from the past, yearning for evidence to fit their intuition, for whom the idea of measuring communication and its effects at all may have seemed a liberation and a vindication of their intuitions.

Let us talk instead to our Dean. This is a version of what we might say.

There have been reviews of the research since the 1980s, most notably from that era by Sanson-Fisher *et al.*[5] At this time, too, Pendleton[6] – one of the great pioneers in the field – set out in a detailed study the various approaches that had been attempted. A few years later, a collection of essays, rigorously constructed and set forward, included an exceptionally helpful overview by Roter.[7] More recently, there has also been something of a recognition that relevant research has included different kinds of approach,[8] although the methodological diversity remains somewhat limited. Rather, the general approach has tended to remain consistent, although individual studies have tried to develop a degree of distinctiveness. Roter pointed out, among other things, that for the '61 separate studies' reported in 80 papers 'we were struck by the fact that so many authors devised their own schemes to analyze interactions rather than use previously developed schemes.' There has been no particular let-up in this area since, although Roter's own scheme (known as Roter's Interaction Analysis System or RIAS[9]) has considerable influence and currency. Roter and her colleagues also looked at 'reported correlates of physician communication with outcome variables – patient satisfaction, recall and compliance.' She concluded:

> Our primary findings . . . [show] significant relations between the outcome variables and almost all of the physician communication groupings.

('Compliance' has in the years since come to seem like an old-fashioned term, of course, and is usually replaced by 'concordance.')

This is a bedrock finding, and the selection of outcome variables is typical of those explored over the years – the findings, too, are representative of what Ong et al.[10] were to sum up in 1995:

> Certain aspects of doctor–patient communication seem to have an influence on patients' behaviour and well-being, for example satisfaction with care, adherence to treatment, recall and understanding of medical information, coping with the disease, quality of life, and even state of health.

This single sentence is bolstered by 18 references in the original, from 1981 onwards, including a further, very brief review (in Stewart and Roter[7]) by Beckman et al. of outcome-based research.[11] Ong et al. discuss this in detail during the course of their review, and confirm that 'some of the frequently used . . . outcomes seem to be indicators of the effectiveness of doctor–patient communication.'

Having said this, it is worth stressing – it's a part of this much-quoted study that tends not to be emphasised – that Ong et al. also state:

> In the past two decades descriptive and experimental research has tried to shed light on the communication process during medical consultations. However, the insight gained from these efforts is limited.

The authors suggest a reason for this:

> This is probably due to the fact that among inter-personal relationships, the doctor–patient relation is one of the most complex ones. It involves interaction between individuals in non-equal positions, is often non-voluntary, concerns issues of vital importance, is therefore emotionally laden, and requires close cooperation.

Anyone who has tried to make sense of communication is likely only to half-agree. It's plausible to think of it as complex, for the reasons given. It is more complex at least than are many other kinds of professional – rather than 'interpersonal' – encounter, such as buying a train-ticket, or ordering a meal in a restaurant. On the other hand, doctor–patient communication, as it is conceived here and throughout most of the literature, has the huge advantage over a great deal of language-based research that it often takes place in a relatively quiet room, frequently with only two speakers. And while one knows what is meant, it's easy enough to quibble about what yardstick for 'complexity' is at stake, and whether our 'inter-personal relationships' with our friends and family are not at least as complex, and a great deal less penetrable from the outside, than our relationships with our doctors and patients.

Nevertheless, although one can cite the occasional negative finding in the literature – for instance, Brown *et al.*[12] found in a randomised controlled trial that their communication skills course simply didn't work – this is one of a small number of papers (that by Griffin *et al.* is another[13]) which recognise that we perhaps know less than we acknowledge.

The selection of outcome measures reflects to a substantial extent the range of elegantly devised and executed experiments set up by Philip Ley in the 1960s and 1970s, which were finally gathered together in 1988.[14] Ley's conclusions are subtle, carefully balanced and conservatively stated, but one can begin to see in them the outlines of what perhaps most of us aim for, at the most basic level – an interaction with a patient which leaves the patient with a clear understanding, a sense of satisfaction, a willingness to co-operate and, as a consequence of all these, the possibility of better health.

'Better health' of course might mean many things – more possibility of a cure in some cases perhaps, or improved morale in others (see, for example, Fallowfield's work with cancer sufferers[15]). The fact that 'cure' is not always the goal of the interaction, in either the short or long term, is something which seems to me to be central to the whole discussion, and I should like to introduce it briefly at this stage, before we go on. Here is how McWhinney[16] expresses it, once more in Stewart and Roter:

> Healing in its deepest sense – the restoration of wholeness – requires a resolution of [spiritual and moral] questions. Healing is not the same as treating or curing. Healing happens to a whole person; that is why we can be cured without being healed, and healed without being cured. A person who remains in anguish of spirit even after physical recovery cannot be said to be healed. Even when cure is not possible, Viktor Frankl (1973) has observed that suffering can be borne more readily if its meaning is understood.

Viktor Frankl was a neurologist and therapist who survived the Nazi death camps. He developed the idea of 'logotherapy' partly in response to his experiences there (although the term itself pre-dates the Nazi era), and to his sense that those who survived the camps were those who were able to see meaning in life, and to discover and maintain a sense of purpose.

> [T]here is also purpose in that life which is almost barren of both creation and enjoyment and which admits of but one possibility of high moral behaviour:

namely, in man's attitude to his existence, and existence restricted by external forces . . . Without suffering and death human life cannot be complete.[17]

At the risk of a degree of bathos, we should observe here in passing that Frankl's concept of understanding is different from the straightforward kind of comprehension with which Ley and Roter are quite reasonably concerned. Are Ley's 'understanding' and 'satisfaction' the same as Frankl's? Simply to ask the question is to see how absurd it is. When process/outcome research asks questions like 'Did you understand?' or 'Are you satisfied?', these are not – and are not intended to be – particularly profound.

However, with Frankl, such concepts are to be answered at a deeper level of our being. Whether this makes them necessarily better or worse is as much a matter of context as of anything else. The foundations of one's being may or may not be altered by contact with the medical profession, but they are unlikely to be particularly stirred by the interest or lack of it that the doctor shows in the fact you have a bit of a cough this morning. Nevertheless, Frankl invites us to ask again: To what extent are the things we can measure the things that matter? And of those things which cannot be measured, what ought we to bother about as educators, or as therapists of the mind or body?

At any rate, the next major landmark in contemporary communication skills – a paper still much referred to, and one with resonance perhaps as much for its committed, slightly defiant tone as for its content – is the so-called Toronto consensus statement, which I have already mentioned.[18] I would like to spend a little time discussing this paper because it remains, probably, not merely the best-known study, but also one whose agenda is still with us.

It begins (again, with echoes from the outcome variables which can be traced back to the 1970s):

> Effective communication between doctor and patient is a central clinical function that cannot be delegated. Most of the essential diagnostic information arises from the interview, and the physician's interpersonal skills also largely determine the patient's satisfaction and compliance and positively influence health outcomes . . . Increasing public dissatisfaction with the medical profession is, in good part, related to deficiencies in clinical communication.

The research cited is gathered under three headings:
- What are the most important facts we already know about doctor–patient communication?
- What are the most important things that could be done now to improve clinical communication by doctors?
- What are the most important unanswered questions and priorities?

What is known – what was known in the early 1990s – is familiar territory. There are, we are told, commonly reported problems with patient concerns being missed by doctors, particularly where they are of a psychological nature. There are disagreements between doctors and patients about what the principal problem is, complaints are not competently dealt with, doctors use 'unclear' language, and so forth. And yet there is evidence that the 'quality of clinical communication is related to positive health outcomes.' Moreover, picking up the central declaration mentioned in the Introduction, although 'Clinical communication skills do not reliably improve from mere experience' they 'can be defined with behavioural criteria and can be reliably taught and assessed.'

With regard to the important things that can be done now, the authors in fact say little, merely listing the kind of thing that is common to all checklists of the era and since (Maguire and Pitceathly's more recent succinct and authoritative summary[19] is mentioned below). So, for example, the statement mentions active listening, empathy, open-ended questions, clear explanations, checking understanding, and so on.

The list of what is not known is intriguing, and raises a good many problems which are still unresolved. They range from the 'specific elements of communication that maximise patient satisfaction, collaborative autonomy, quality of life, enhancement of coping, and adaptation and recovery or rehabilitation while minimising conflict and litigation' to the issue of 'physician, patient, family and practice variables', to how 'needs and practice vary in the course of continuing clinical care', and include the relationship between ethics and communication. The paper also raises the issue of what the best teaching methodologies might be.

So, in summary, the teaching of communication can be achieved, it is a goal worth trying to achieve, 'good' communication can be defined, but there are also a lot of unresolved issues. These are the facts that are claimed, but the tone is no less important. There is an uncompromising belief in the value of good communication, and in the virtues of teaching it, and a belief based straightforwardly – almost pugnaciously – on research evidence which centres around measurable aspects of behaviour.

There have been other reviews since this time. That of Aspegren[20] is listed on the Best Evidence Medical Education (BEME) website.[21] The phrase 'best evidence' is used by many to draw attention to the fact that there are many aspects of medical education which are not, in principle, amenable to the kinds of precise investigation associated with randomised controlled trials. Aspegren's rationale was that:

> Since this training is both costly and time-consuming, there is a need to collect
> the present knowledge in the field of communication skills teaching and learning
> in order to make it easier for teachers and curricular committees to find the
> pertinent information on the subject.

There is here, incidentally, an implicit assumption that 'communication skills'
are necessarily an addition to the curriculum. And the discipline is of course
particularly vulnerable to financial scrutiny because so much of it must
be done in very small groups, in order to give individuals the opportunity
for proper practice. This is true of a great deal of medical education, where
observation and practice are central to the whole enterprise, but the need for
communication is – and has been perceived as being – less obvious. To which
one might argue (if context is all) that it need not be quite so much of an add-on
as all that – that it can be learned and practised in the context of the ward, or of
the surgery. Equally, clinical skills can be practised where the ostensible subject
is communication, and the result of this kind of contextualisation can easily be
a more economical approach than one might imagine.

Aspegren identified 180 papers in all, and from these he selected 31 randomised studies, 38 open effect studies and 14 descriptive studies as fulfilling
'"high" and "medium" quality criteria' according to a well-defined set of
criteria developed in Sanson-Fisher et al.[5] He lists 'ten methods' which were
found for the measurement of communication skills (see Table 2.3). The list
makes fascinating reading, reflecting both common practice in evaluation
and, due to the inevitable vagueness and subjectivity implicit in many of the
methodologies, reflecting no less clearly the difficulties in obtaining valid and
reliable evaluations.

Aspegren's findings are very definite, although by this time (in the late
1990s) what he says acts as formal confirmation of what people – at any rate
people on the right side of the fence – had begun to take pretty much as the
accepted wisdom. This was that 'There is overwhelming evidence for a positive
effect of communication skills training' and, later, 'The main finding of the
review is that there is overwhelming proof that communication skills in the
patient–doctor relationship can be taught and are learned', although he also
recognises that because 'At present, there is no satisfactory integrated theory
on the physician–patient relationship . . . training courses are generally ad
hoc.' This last point can be compared with Roter's sense of disappointment that
individual researchers have tended to build their own systems rather than work
with and develop what is already in the literature.

Table 2.3 How communication skills were measured in the various studies[20]

Ten methods were found:

1. Course evaluation. The participants have stated their opinions about the usefulness, etc. of the training.
2. Written report by the student of the contents, etc. of an interview.
3. Cognitive testing of the knowledge about medical interviewing.
4. Self-rating scales.
5. Psychometric tests of some kind, which are assumed to correlate with communication skills.
6. Direct observation by an external observer, most often using a rating scale.
7. Video- or audiotaped interviews rated by an independent and trained observer using a rating scale and/or global assessment.
8. OSCE examination.
9. Patient's rating of the student's performance, often with the aid of a rating scale.
10. Patient health outcome.

The most thorough of all studies of this kind – studies which centre, that is, on evidence-based lists of skills – are the two books by Kurtz, Silverman and Draper[22,23] (the first two named share first authorship status for both books, but I list them here alphabetically). These texts, and the 'Calgary–Cambridge' approach in which they originate, are exhaustively researched, and have been developed over 15 years or so. They are also in many respects rather misrepresented, with readers seeming often to take the list of skills which they elaborate as being the sum of the method.[24] In fact, however, the authors talk of three 'types of communication skills', as shown in Table 2.4.

Table 2.4 Types of communication skills and how they interrelate; from Kurtz *et al.*[22,23]

1. **Content skills** – *what healthcare professionals communicate* – the substance of their questions and responses, the information that they gather and give, and the treatments they discuss.

2. **Process skills** – *how they do it* – the ways in which they communicate with patients and how they go about discovering the history or providing information, the verbal and non-verbal skills that they use, how they develop the relationship with the patient, and the way they organise and structure communication.

3. **Perceptual skills** – *what they are thinking and feeling* – their internal decision-making, clinical reasoning and problem-solving skills, their attitudes and intentions, values and beliefs, their awareness of feelings and thoughts about the patient, about the illness and about other issues that may be concerning them, and their awareness of their own self-concept and confidence, and of their own biases and distractions.

A list of the 71 process skills themselves is easily available online.[25] They look, all strung out like this, a bit formidable. There are, well, rather a lot, and there is a great deal of apparent category mixing in the skills. Most linguists, for instance, would have trouble putting 'uses open and closed questioning techniques' as a concept at the same linguistic level as 'organising explanation' (or for that matter 'language') – partly because an explanation is bigger than an open question, perhaps, but also because of that mix of objects (language), methods (techniques) and outcomes (organisation). Nevertheless, the general approach is unquestionably useful, and the list is an immensely helpful, pragmatic device.

Having said this, anyone interested in the field should be familiar with the books rather than the skills checklist which they have given rise to. Indeed, the authors point out, 'It is important to emphasise that content, process and perceptual skills are inextricably linked and cannot be considered in isolation.' However, the authors also acknowledge that 'this book [*Teaching and Learning Communication Skills in Medicine*] and its companion focus primarily on process skills', the logic here being that 'particular content skills, such as the questions that constitute the review of systems or that need to be asked to investigate a specific problem . . . are well described in many textbooks', and 'The same can be said of the clinical reasoning and medical problem-solving aspects of perceptual skills.'

The difficulty is probably that very complex category of perceptual skills which, precisely because they are not the primary focus of attention, are permitted relatively little space for discussion. Given the amount of attention that is afforded the concept of 'attitude' in the present professional climate, for example, it seems strange to see it listed merely as one of a number of 'perceptual skills.'

If Kurtz, Silverman and Draper are the most thorough analysts of process skills and their contexts, then Maguire and Pitceathly[19] are the most succinct. Maguire is an immensely experienced worker in the communication skills field, particularly in oncology,[26] and is himself a contributor of influential research, so that the skills he identifies come with the additional force of experience. With regard to 'skills needed to perform key tasks', Maguire and Pitceathly talk in the familiar and traditional terms, for example:

> Establish eye contact at the beginning of the consultation and maintain it at reasonable intervals to show interest. Encourage patients to be exact about the sequence in which their problems occurred; ask for dates of key events and about patients' perceptions and feelings . . .

And so on. This is, at the time of writing, probably the single paper of choice to give a doctor who doesn't understand what communication skills are, or who needs affirmation that they matter.

One final point needs to be made in this section. The Toronto statement drew attention to the fact that we knew little, in the late 1980s and early 1990s, about how communication varied with the clinical setting, with the process of the illness, and so on. On the whole, this remains true, although Roter in particular has provided us with a description of various settings, ranging for example from emergency medicine[27] to sexual health[28] to veterinary medicine.[29]

However, something of an exception can be made for communication in cancer, and the special consideration in serious illness of breaking bad news (BBN) – or, as it is sometimes called, 'significant news' – has been the subject of very substantial concern.

Maguire's work has already been mentioned briefly. (Maguire and Faulkner published a number of studies on this topic in the *British Medical Journal* as far back as 1988. One of these has already been mentioned in passing, but see also, for example, their two papers on 'How to communicate with cancer patients.'[30,31]) Another individual who should be mentioned in this context is Fallowfield, for a series of empirical studies which form a significant part of the educational base. Her starting point is the simple fact that 'Doctors and nurses usually talk and listen to patients more than they perform any other single medical or nursing procedure.'[32] Fallowfield *et al.*[33] is one of the few persuasive accounts of a randomised controlled trial in the area, reporting as it does on the results of a trial involving 160 doctors who were randomised into groups that received 'A, written feedback followed by course, B, course only, C, written feedback only, or D, control.' The results were in one sense appropriately encouraging: 'training courses significantly improve key communication skills.' However, as with so many evaluations of this sort, one is left a little puzzled. Most well-designed and well-delivered courses work, in any discipline. People who believe otherwise really shouldn't be in education. What actually matters is the details of the programme. (Incidentally, Fallowfield is also joint author of an excellent recent review of what she calls 'sad, bad and difficult news',[34] one which supersedes the other major review article in the area, by Ptacek and Eberhardt.[35])

The public context

Well then, Dean, such is the state of the evidence. I have, I acknowledge, included a few small caveats here and there, but most people accept that the evidence is robust. Have I convinced you?

No? Then let me talk a little about the public arena. Ours is a medical school at the cutting edge, is it not? We wish to reflect the requirements of our governing bodies, and beyond them our government, and beyond that the patients whom we exist to serve, and whose expectations are – well, I refer you to the first audience in the previous section. Ours is a world of talk and mutual respect.

So, then, the evidence that I have cited is the evidence which has set the mood, and behind it is the more public, more political face – a recognition that in western society we try to sustain a kind of democracy in our dealings with our fellow citizens, both professionally and privately. There is a recognition that no particular set of views is paramount, or alternatively that the patient's wishes are paramount where proper alternatives have been described, and so on.

Part of this political level of debate concerns itself with such things as the link between communication, formal complaints and litigation. Levinson *et al.*, for example, argue that 'Surprisingly, the differences between sued and never-sued physicians are not explained by their quality of care or their chart documentation.'[36] Hickson *et al.* have reached similar conclusions.[37,38] Levinson *et al.* go on to state:

> Patient dissatisfaction is critical. The combination of a bad outcome and patient dissatisfaction is a recipe for litigation. When faced with a bad outcome, patients and families are more likely to sue a physician if they feel the physician was not caring and compassionate. Breakdowns in communication between physicians and patients lead to patient anger and dissatisfaction and possible litigation. Conversely, effective communication enhances patient satisfaction and health outcomes.

And with this last sentence we are back on familiar territory. Incidentally, Levinson and her colleagues are careful to emphasise that their findings and the implications held for primary care, but not in fact for other disciplines, specifically surgery:

> The study identifies specific and teachable communication behaviors associated with fewer malpractice claims for primary care physicians. Physicians can use these findings as they seek to improve communication and decrease malpractice risk. Malpractice insurers can use this information to guide malpractice risk prevention and education for primary care physicians, but should not assume that it is appropriate to teach similar behaviors to other specialty groups.

Unsurprisingly, given the sheer volume of argument, public and political documents have followed suit. Everywhere in the western world, at least, we have seen what one might call the routinisation of communication skills, and of related areas.

In the UK, *Tomorrow's Doctors*,[39] published by the General Medical Council with the explicit aim of driving undergraduate medical education, was arguing in its first iteration, in 1993, that good communication was a core skill for undergraduates to master. And if that statement appeared a little daring in those days, more was on offer by the early years of the present century. The 2003 (and current) issue of this central document lists 27 elements of curricular content (numbered 11 to 37 within the document), of which communication is permitted four elements, with some offered a degree of detail (*see* Table 2.5).

Table 2.5 *Tomorrow's Doctors* – communication skills[39]

20. Graduates must be able to communicate clearly, sensitively and effectively with patients and their relatives, and colleagues from a variety of health and social care professions. Clear communication will help them carry out their various roles, including clinician, team member, team leader and teacher.

21. Graduates must know that some individuals use different methods of communication, for example, Deafblind Manual and British Sign Language.

22. Graduates must be able to do the following.

   a. Communicate effectively with individuals regardless of their social, cultural or ethnic backgrounds, or their disabilities.

   b. Communicate with individuals who cannot speak English, including working with interpreters.

23. Students must have opportunities to practise communicating in different ways, including spoken, written and electronic methods. There should also be guidance about how to cope in difficult circumstances. Some examples are listed below.

   a. Breaking bad news.

   b. Dealing with difficult and violent patients.

   c. Communicating with people with mental illness, including cases where patients have special difficulties in sharing how they feel and think with doctors.

   d. Communicating with and treating patients with severe mental or physical disabilities.

   e. Helping vulnerable patients.

The range of non-clinical areas in general has developed, in fact, to include such matters as basic teaching skills, for instance:

24. Graduates must understand the principles of education as they are applied to medicine. They will be familiar with a range of teaching and learning techniques and must recognise their obligation to teach colleagues. They

must understand the importance of audit and appraisal in identifying learning needs for themselves and their colleagues.

Such documents, as we saw in the previous chapter, take their shape from the transient socio-political dialogues of the day. The meanings of words depend on the context in which they are uttered. 'I wish the ground would swallow me up' means different things spoken by a depressed patient and the new secretary who can't find the file her boss has asked her for. It's a sign of the times that only about six or so – depending on what you include and exclude – of the 25 sub-headings in which 'curricular content' is described are straightforwardly clinical, with the balance including time management, reflective learning, the relationship between the doctor and society, and the like. To put it another way, there are roughly 8 clinical column inches out of 28.

The willingness to endorse this kind of variety hints at the enthusiasm for a broad-based training, sketched but not explicitly justified in the 1993 document's references to Special Study Modules (SSMs), which need not be medical. Now the expectation is for these SSMs, relabelled as 'Student-Selected Components' (SSCs), to occupy 25–33% of the curriculum, with at least two-thirds of them being medical. Even then, within these two-thirds one may study the traditionally 'soft' areas of behavioural sciences, or the even softer medical humanities. By simple arithmetic, this might therefore allow a student to base as much as one-ninth of their curriculum on completely 'non-medical' subjects, provided that they can be demonstrated to hit a number of general targets mentioned in the document, such as developing research skills.

At post-qualification level, the situation is the same. *Good Medical Practice*[40] argues for communication skills. It states that 'Good communication between patients and doctors is essential to effective care and relationships of trust', before going on to specify that this involves listening, information giving and the like. The British Medical Association (BMA)[41] describes it as a core skill:

> [Communication] is an essential competency, which health professionals must have . . . communicative and interpersonal skills are technical skills which can be learned, and the doctor who lacks them can be said to be lacking in technique, in the same way as the doctor who lacks clinical knowledge.

This is a helpful quotation, couched as it is in terms of an explicit identity with other skills, something as immediately pertinent as that of taking a blood pressure – a statement that 'communication' is the same, not different.

Since then, the tragedy at the Bristol Royal Infirmary in the UK, when it appeared that children who were undergoing complex heart surgery were not appropriately managed, has had a major impact on training in the UK. The subsequent Bristol Royal Infirmary (BRI) Enquiry[42] highlighted communication among a range of other highly pertinent factors as part of 'broadening the notion of clinical competence.' The Enquiry recommended that 'Greater priority than at present should be given to . . . skills in communicating with patients and with colleagues.'

Similarly in the UK, as part of the initiative known as Modernising Medical Careers, communication skills are treated as a generic skill.[43] There have also been changes to the Membership examinations for the Royal Colleges – not only with regard to general practice, which is at the ostensibly, touchy-feely, discursive end of the medical spectrum, and where an examination of consultation skills (rather than communication skills) has been established for some years, but also with regard to the more traditionally scientific disciplines. There have been changes to PACES (Practical Assessment of Clinical Examination Skills),[44] for example, the examination for membership of the Royal College of Physicians, in which the examination component is in fact called 'communication skills and ethics', and that for membership of the Royal College of Surgeons,[45] which includes as criteria just the kind of behavioural checklist with which we are already familiar.

With regard to North America, for example, I have already mentioned the work of Project Professionalism in the USA (*see* Chapter 1, page 6). In the USA, just as in the UK, there has been fallout from the BRI Enquiry and the Shipman affair.[46] One of the drivers has been the discovery of criminal and sometimes murderous behaviour, as in the Michael Swango case.[47]

Thus the Liaison Committee on Medical Education (which accredits North American MD programmes) was stating in the mid-1990s that:

> there must be specific instruction and evaluation of [communication] skills as they relate to physician responsibilities, including communication with patients, families, colleagues and other health professionals.

Training in communication is widespread in North America, at least according to self-reports, with most schools using either the Calgary–Cambridge approach or SEGUE.[48] Similarly, the US Medical Licensing Examination (USMLE) added in 2004 'an assessment of communication and other interpersonal skills; and an assessment of proficiency in spoken English',[49] and by 1998 the Association of American Medical Colleges had incorporated a range of elements traditionally regarded as 'non-clinical' as essential learning objectives.[50] This included communication skills:

The ability to communicate effectively, both orally and in writing, with patients, patients' families, colleagues, and others with whom physicians must exchange information in carrying out their responsibilities.

This comes under the sub-heading 'Physicians must be skilful.' Indeed, physicians must be – with the sub-headings listed in this order – *altruistic, knowledgeable, skilful* and *dutiful*. 'Altruism' includes mention of a specific recognition of a major preoccupation in the USA:

. . . the threats to medical professionalism posed by the conflicts of interest inherent in various financial and organizational arrangements for the practice of medicine.

The mention of 'duty' as an abstract concept is also of interest, in the context of my earlier remarks. You may feel either that the description of the dutiful physician is too wide-ranging to be of value, or that it captures well what the 'good doctor' we searched for in the previous chapter is like:

Physicians must feel obliged to collaborate with other health professionals and to use systematic approaches for promoting, maintaining and improving the health of individuals and populations. They must be knowledgeable about the risk factors for disease and injury, must understand how to utilize disease and injury prevention practices in the care of individual patients, must promote healthy behaviors through counseling individual patients and their families and public education and action, must actively support traditional public health practices in their communities, and must be advocates for improving access to care for everyone, especially those who are members of traditionally underserved populations. They must understand the economic, psychological, occupational, social and cultural factors that contribute to the development and/ or perpetuation of conditions that impair health. In caring for individual patients, they must apply the principles of evidence-based medicine and cost effectiveness in making decisions about the utilization of limited medical resources. They must be committed to working collaboratively with other physicians; other health care professionals (including administrators of hospitals, health care organizations, and systems of care); and individuals representing a wide variety of community agencies. As members of a team addressing individual or population-based health care issues, they must be willing both to provide leadership when appropriate and to defer to the leadership of others when indicated. They must acknowledge and respect the roles of other health professionals in providing needed services to individual patients, populations or communities.

This does no more than hint at the explosion of interest in, and public sensitivity to, communication skills in healthcare. Nursing, struggling with an even more suspiciously caring and vapid image than general practice, is sophisticated here in terms of its research and its public statements. Perhaps more unexpected straws in the wind are offered by both dentistry and veterinary science, which have taken the plunge and recognised the importance of communication (an initial conference on Communication in Veterinary Medicine, said to be the first in the world, was held in 2004[51]). In both of these professions, apart from anything else there is a frankly high risk of ridicule of the very idea that communication matters. Thus in the UK, with regard to the former, the General Dental Council's guiding statement on undergraduate dentistry[52] states that:

> the dental graduate must be able to:
>
> communicate effectively with patients, their families and associates, and with other health professionals involved in their care.

And with regard to veterinary medicine, among the 'Day 1 Competencies' required of the 'new veterinary graduate', the Royal College of Veterinary Science[53] states that they must be able to:

> Communicate effectively with clients, the lay public, professional colleagues and responsible authorities; listen effectively and respond sympathetically to clients and others, using language in a form appropriate to the audience and the context.

All of this, then, is what we might say as we defend the discipline, or ask for better resourcing. In a nutshell, we can express it as follows.

Dear Dean, We can prove good communication skills are teachable, and that they make a difference to patient satisfaction, and to patient health. We can show that they will keep the doctor away from the lawyers. You will already be aware that the GMC and all manner of such people think we should be teaching them. And it fits in with the kind of society we live in, frankly.

Please renew my contract. Just the three years will do, actually. After that I'm going to try the same line of argument somewhere that will really appreciate me. Your loyal servant.

And this is our inheritance.

References

1 Eliot TS. Ash Wednesday. In: *Complete Poems and Plays.* London: Faber; 2004.
2 http://news.bbc.co.uk/1/low/health/1952712.stm (accessed 14 February 2006).
3 http://healthcaremonster.com/articles/bedside (accessed 20 February 2006).
4 Smithers A. Medical education is heading for disaster. *Independent,* 19 September 2002.
5 Sanson-Fisher R, Fairburn S, Maguire P. Teaching skills in communication to medical students – a critical view of the methodology. *Med Educ.* 1981; **15:** 33–7.
6 Pendleton D, Hasler J, editors. *Doctor–Patient Communication.* London: Academic Press; 1983.
7 Roter D. Which facets of communication have strong effects on outcome? A meta-analysis. In: Stewart M, Roter D, editors. *Communicating With Medical Patients.* Newbury Park, CA: Sage; 1989. pp. 183–96.
8 Bower P, Gask L, May C *et al.* Domains of consultation research in primary care. *Patient Educ Counsel.* 2001; **45:** 3–11.
9 Roter D. The Roter method of interaction process analysis; www.rias.org/manual (accessed 17 January 2007).
10 Ong LM, de Haes JC, Hoos AM *et al.* Doctor–patient communication: a review of the literature. *Soc Sci Med.* 1995; **40:** 903–18.
11 Beckman H, Kaplan S, Frankel R. Outcome-based research on doctor–patient communication: a review. In: Stewart M, Roter D, editors. *Communicating With Medical Patients.* Newbury Park, CA: Sage; 1989. pp. 223–7.
12 Brown JB, Boles M, Mullooly JP *et al.* Effect of clinical communication skills training on patient satisfaction. A randomized controlled trial. *Ann Intern Med.* 1999; **131:** 822–9.
13 Griffin SJ, Kinmonth A-L, Veltman MWM *et al.* Effect on health-related outcomes of interventions to alter the interaction between patients and practitioners: a systematic review of trials. *Ann Fam Med.* 2004; **2:** 595–608.
14 Ley P. *Communicating With Patients: improving communication satisfaction and compliance.* Cheltenham: Stanley Thornes; 1988.
15 Fallowfield L, Jenkins V, Farewell V *et al.* Efficacy of a Cancer Research UK communication skills training model for oncologists: a randomised trial. *Lancet.* 2002; **359:** 650–56.
16 McWhinney IR. The need for a transformed clinical method. In: Stewart M, Roter D, editors. *Communicating With Medical Patients.* Newbury Park, CA: Sage; 1989. pp. 25–40.
17 Frankl V (Winston R, Winston C, trans.). *The Doctor and the Soul: from psychotherapy to logotherapy.* Harmondsworth: Penguin; 1973.
18 Simpson M, Buckman R, Stewart M *et al.* Doctor–patient communication: the Toronto consensus statement. *BMJ.* 1991; **303:** 1385–7.
19 Maguire P, Pitceathly C. Key communication skills and how to acquire them. *BMJ.* 2002; **325:** 697, 700.

20 Aspegren K. Teaching and learning communication skills in medicine: a review with quality grading of articles. *Med Teacher.* 1999; **21:** 563–70.

21 Best Evidence Medical Education (BEME); www.bemecollaboration.org (accessed 18 January 2007).

22 Silverman J, Kurtz S, Draper J. *Skills for Communicating with Patients.* Oxford: Radcliffe Medical Press; 1998.

23 Kurtz S, Silverman J, Draper J. *Teaching and Learning Communication Skills in Medicine.* Oxford: Radcliffe Medical Press; 1998.

24 Silverman J. The Calgary–Cambridge guides: the 'teenage years'. *Clin Teacher.* 2007; **4:** 87–93.

25 Cheek B. www.gp-training.net/training/communication_skills/calgary/calgary. pdf (accessed 29 October 2007).

26 Maguire P, Faulkner A. How to improve the counselling skills of doctors and nurses in cancer care. *BMJ.* 1988; **297:** 847–9.

27 Farmer SA, Roter DL, Higginson IJ. Chest pain: communication of symptoms and history in a London emergency department. *Patient Educ Counsel.* 2006; **63:** 138–44.

28 Roter DL, Knowles N, Somerfield M *et al.* Routine communication in sexually transmitted disease clinics: an observational study. *Am J Public Health.* 1990; **80:** 605–6.

29 Shaw JR, Adams CL, Bonnett BN *et al.* Use of the Roter interaction analysis system to analyze veterinarian–client–patient communication in companion animal practice. *J Am Vet Med Assoc.* 2004; **225:** 222–9.

30 Maguire P, Faulkner A. Communicate with cancer patients. 1. Handling bad news and difficult questions. *BMJ.* 1988; **297:** 907–9.

31 Maguire P, Faulkner A. Communicate with cancer patients. 2. Handling uncertainty, collusion and denial. *BMJ.* 1988; **297:** 972–4.

32 Fallowfield L, Jenkins V. Effective communication skills are the key to good cancer care. *Eur J Cancer.* 1999; **35:** 1592–7.

33 Fallowfield L, Jenkins V, Farewell V *et al.* Efficacy of a Cancer Research UK communication skills training model for oncologists: a randomised trial. *Lancet.* 2002; **359:** 650–56.

34 Fallowfield L, Jenkins V. Communicating sad, bad and difficult news in medicine. *Lancet.* 2004; **363:** 312–19.

35 Ptacek JT, Eberhardt T. Breaking bad news: a review of the literature. *JAMA.* 1996; **276:** 496–502.

36 Levinson W, Roter DL, Mullooly JP *et al.* Physician–patient communication: the relationship with malpractice claims among primary care physicians and surgeons. *JAMA.* 1997; **277:** 553–9.

37 Hickson GB, Clayton EW, Githens PB *et al.* Factors that prompted families to file medical malpractice claims following perinatal injuries. *JAMA.* 1992; **267:** 1359–63.

38 Hickson GB, Clayton EW, Entman SS *et al.* Obstetricians' prior malpractice experience and patients' satisfaction with care. *JAMA.* **272:** 1583–7.

39 General Medical Council. *Tomorrow's Doctors.* London: General Medical Council;
    2003; www.gmc-uk.org/education/undergraduate/tomdoc.pdf (accessed
    23 January 2007).

40 General Medical Council. *Good Medical Practice.* London: General Medical Council;
    2006; www.gmc-uk.org/guidance/good_medical_practice/index.asp (accessed
    23 January 2007).

41 British Medical Association. *Communication Skills and Continuing Professional
    Development.* London: British Medical Association; 1998.

42 The Bristol Royal Infirmary Enquiry, July 2001; www.bristol-inquiry.org.uk/
    final_report/report/index.htm (accessed 19 January 2007).

43 Foundation Programme Committee, Academy of Royal Medical Colleges;
    www.mmc.nhs.uk/download_files/Curriculum-for-the-foundation-years-in-
    postgraduate-education-and-training.pdf (accessed 2 April 2007).

44 Royal Colleges of Physicians of the United Kingdom; www.mrcpuk.org/plain/
    PACES.html (accessed 13 March 2007).

45 Royal College of Surgeons of England; www.rcseng.ac.uk/exams/docs/mrcs/
    candid_comm.pdf (accessed 13 March 2007).

46 The Shipman Inquiry; www.the-shipman-inquiry.org.uk (accessed 13 March
    2007).

47 Stewart JB. *Blind Eye: how the medical establishment let a doctor get away with
    murder.* New York: Simon and Schuster; 1999.

48 Makoul G. Communication skills education in medical school and beyond. *Student
    JAMA.* 2003; **289:** 93.

49 Papadakis M. The 2-step clinical skills examination. *NEJM.* 2004; **350:** 1703–5.

50 Association of American Medical Colleges. Learning objectives for medical
    education; www.aamc.org/meded/msop/msop1.pdf (accessed 21 February
    2007).

51 American Association of Veterinary Medicine; www.avma.org/onlnews/javma/
    nov04/041115m.asp (accessed 31 August 2007).

52 General Dental Council, UK; www.gdc-uk.org/NR/rdonlyres/4B6221BD-6224-
    415A-A0C3-8AD241DE249D/15158/first_five_years_2002.pdf (accessed 13
    March 2007).

53 Royal College of Veterinary Surgeons, UK; www.rcvs.org.uk/shared_asp_files/
    uploadedfiles/2d23a15d-842b-4838-9ca2-9ae68d9a6998_ems_apr_06.pdf
    (accessed 14 March 2007).

CHAPTER 3

Language, rhetoric and the discourse community

. . . experimentation has always been an activity undertaken with, or on behalf of, others. It is a socially established and co-operative human activity, like building a house, selling insurance, managing a business, playing football, etc. The scientific laboratory is a place where people meet to report, to witness, to agree and disagree, to negotiate, and to interact, as well as a place where hypotheses are tested . . . the social role of the laboratory and lecture as scenes for the operation of the experimental method have been prominent since the seventeenth century . . . the truth or otherwise of some general theory might be accessible only to God, but the reliability of the report of an experiment . . . was a matter of social credibility. The skills of an experimenter such as Robert Hooke could be, and were, bought; but those who witnessed his experiments were required to have social standing in the community if they wished others to believe their reports . . . It is as though the social fabric determines what will be believed and accepted.

(B Gower, *Scientific Method* [1])

What's aught but as 'tis valued?

(W Shakespeare, *Troilus and Cressida*, II.ii.51 [2])

Introduction

We have our inheritance indeed, then. However, I would like to subject it to scrutiny, not least because communication skills is – 'is still', I almost wrote – a fashionable subject, and it is at just such a point, before fashion gives way to suspicion, that we should take a long hard look at the question of how robust the discipline is, and how easily therefore it will absorb criticism.

We all know, referring back to our hypothetical Dean of the last chapter, that it can seem very difficult to get communication to the top of anyone's agenda. However, we help no one – least of all ourselves, in the long run – if we are not entirely clear about what we can claim, and what we cannot claim.

There are three things I would therefore like to do in this chapter and the next. The first is to look more closely at the idea that nothing happens in isolation – that political statements, and research itself, take place within an existing context of debate. I want, that is, to introduce the concept of the 'discourse community' briefly. The second issue, which I shall explore at greater length, is to look in the light of this at the function of the behavioural checklist. And the third issue is to consider the notion of 'communicative competence.' The first and third of these concepts are familiar to linguists.

Academic medicine: the discourse community

My suggestion in the opening paragraph, that 'we' should seek to be certain about what we can claim, is obviously a political statement, a statement about strategy – and I have already remarked in passing on the slightly evangelical tone of the Toronto statement. There has long been an element of proselytisation in the field. Indeed, communication skills is a perfect example of a discipline where the name of the game is persuasion – persuasion, to be sure, through what is intended to look like the unbiased presentation of conventionally reached scientific conclusions, but persuasion for all that. And in consequence, there has been little discussion about how research into communication ought to be approached, and whether, in particular, the conventions of the randomised controlled trial are appropriate.

The view that science takes place in a social context is a commonplace. Indeed, there is what one might almost call a traditional view that science over-states its objectivity – a tradition often presented as more radical than it is, and sometimes as downright anti-science. And at its worst, it is downright tiresome. On the other hand, the best of the tradition is excellent, much of it dating from the profound, and profoundly provocative, work of David Bloor[3] and colleagues in Edinburgh in the 1970s. The study of the sociology of science has since been carried forward in a variety of different and often competing ways.[4,5]

All this line of enquiry shares a recognition, in other words, that science is *fabricated* rather than discovered ('fabrication' is Chalmers' word, in his illuminating review of the issues[6]). The implication is not that there is anything underhand at work, but merely that the relationship between science and 'fact' is more complex than non-scientists think.

Part of the way that science is constructed – or that academic knowledge is constructed, one might say more loosely – is through the medium of the relevant *discourse community*. The above quotation from Gower shows just such a community in action, as indeed does the kind of interaction that takes place at any modern conference. The term 'discourse community' itself was originally coined by Nystrand,[7] but I shall follow Swales' account.[8] He proposes 'six defining characteristics', as follows:

1   a broadly agreed set of common public goals
2   mechanisms of intercommunication
3   participatory mechanisms primarily to provide information and feedback
4   utilisation and possession of one or more genres in the communicative furtherance of its aims
5   specific lexis
6   a threshold level of members with a suitable degree of relevant content and discoursal expertise.

Swales points out that 'those interested in discourse communities have typically sited their discussions within academic contexts, thus possibly creating a false impression that such communities are only to be associated with intellectual paradigms or scholarly cliques.' To make the point that this is not so, he illustrates his definition with reference to a philately club. Rather neatly, he recounts (Swales is both a linguist and a keen philatelist) how he entered into a debate about some abstruse problem through the pages of a relevant magazine, adducing linguistic evidence to support his case, only to be told by another correspondent that he was being 'too clever by half.' The point is well taken. To be a member of the community is to play the game by the community's rules, and to accept the rules of evidence which pertain.

For our purposes, however, the relevant community is indeed academic. It is fairly clear how the community of 'academic medicine' would meet Swales' criteria listed above (perhaps apart from the reference to 'genre', which has a technical meaning in language study, although one not too far removed from the ordinary language meaning).

The 'public goals' are the furtherance of medical science, improvements in patient care and the like. 'Mechanisms of intercommunication', 'participatory mechanisms' and 'genres' all include things like conference papers, journal articles, emails between scholars and so on, and the 'threshold level' of members is self-explanatory. With regard to 'specific lexis' – the vocabulary of the field – this is one area where the selective nature of membership can be most clearly demonstrated.

In part, this is a matter of using jargon to indicate membership of the discipline – the doctor who talks of 'ca bronchus' to colleagues rather than 'lung cancer', or 'tympanic membrane' rather than 'eardrum', for instance. This kind of signalling is identical to what one observes in teenage slang – saying 'ca bronchus' is no different from saying 'wicked' to mean 'good.' Specific pieces of lexis range from the careful, formal definitions of technical terms such as 'significant' to the way that buzzwords come and go ('governance'), to abbreviations ('RCT') and even metaphors – 'gold standard' being a very common one in academic medicine. The ability to use these terms correctly – that is, in accordance with conventions – affirms one's membership of the group.

However, this kind of issue pervades more things than one is immediately aware of. One of the first things I noticed in writing academic medicine after years in language and education, for example, was two crucial ways in which my writing habits were consistently changed by editors and reviewers. One was that the typically tentative claims I made for research findings (typical, that is, of the humanities and social sciences) were made more certain. Where I might write 'This suggests that X is the case . . .', editors routinely corrected this to 'This shows that X is the case . . .', for example – I confess that this still makes me feel uncomfortable. And my frequent use of the present tense to report findings in the Results section of my papers was uniformly rendered into the past tense. Thus 'A number of participants state that X . . .' became 'A number of participants stated that X . . .'. The first point, incidentally, is touched on by Hyland,[9] who explored the way that writers report on the work of other authors. (And in this sentence, you will see that I have used 'is touched on' rather than 'was touched on', and 'explored' rather than, say, 'measured.') Looking at a cross-section of disciplines, not including medicine, Hyland found that:

> Verbs such as *argue* (100% of cases), *suggest* (82%) and *study* (70%) were favoured by the social sciences/humanities writers, while *report* (82%), *describe* (70%) and *show* (55%) occurred mainly in the science/engineering articles.

Without this basic understanding of the language that the community uses, one will not get published, for example – or, as happened to me, the quid pro quo for publication is conformity to group norms.

However, there are other relevant issues. Research consists, in large part, of a dialogue between researchers, agreeing and disagreeing, seeking ways forward, positioning their own work in relation to that of others, and so on. And for our purposes, it consists among other things of the background noise of researchers arguing for something they value, or for curriculum space, or for their own careers. There is a substantial research industry in this area, it should be mentioned. Swales and Hyland have already been cited, but there are many others.[10–12] Aspects of the debate sometimes also surface in the medical press. Horton, for example, speaks of 'the manipulation of language to convince the reader of the likely truth of a result.'[13]

The questions raised by this kind of discussion are profound, and I explore them in greater detail in the companion volume to this book. For the moment, I want simply to ask for recognition that many central questions about medical communication are matters of political strategy, and that when I discuss research I am talking of research in context, and talking therefore of members of the discourse community engaging in the real world, and seeking to persuade, rather than of the scientist in his or her public guise, the self-effacing reporter of objective truths. And these key questions are as follows. What will the discourse community accept as evidence? Should I change the nature of the evidence I collect to suit the community, or persuade the discourse community to change its views about what evidence is?

For what it is worth, my own view is that those of us who work in medical communication try to conform too much. I consider that we would be better advised to develop research strategies that work for the discipline, and that draw therefore not purely on quantitative research – and, for that matter, look also beyond the loose aggregate of techniques that usually attract the term 'qualitative research' as that term is used in healthcare. We should look, therefore, towards an understanding of clinical communication which is driven by an understanding of the nature of language and communication in general, and should look therefore at the application of methodologies which permit sophisticated description.

Not to do this – but to continue with the familiar because the community understands us better – is rather like an astronomer deciding to use a telescope to look at the birds in the back garden, because telescopes are powerful things, that's what astronomers use to bring things closer, and it's what he's used to. And anyway, how else can he persuade the Chief Astronomer that the robins have come again this year? In the end, if we can return to the Dean of the previous chapter, do we offer him the clumsy apparatus of an inappropriate telescope, or do we say 'Just look'?

The general and the specific

The strong version of the case for clinical communication can be summarised in a couple of sentences.

We have the evidence to demonstrate the value of what we teach, and the vocabulary to give a shape and structure to communication. In that sense, we have answers to two central questions. Firstly, why do you teach? And secondly, what do you teach?

The question is whether this case is overstated.

We might, for example, begin with Ong *et al.*, whose review was cited earlier (reference 10 in Chapter 2). They conclude (I should point out, since I shall be talking about 'communicative competence' below, that Ong *et al.* do not use the term 'communicative' in any particularly theoretical way):

> In summary, background variables [for which see below] seem to influence communicative behaviors, these behaviors in their turn have an effect on patient outcomes. Whether all of these variables are in fact related to each other, and if so, in what way, should be studied empirically.
>
> A theory relating these different variables could result in the development of interventions which improve communication in the medical setting, the doctor–patient relationship, and patient outcomes. In this review we have tried to set the framework for such a theory.

What would such a theory look like? The framework is clear enough, at least in its broad outlines, and is presented by Ong *et al.* as follows:

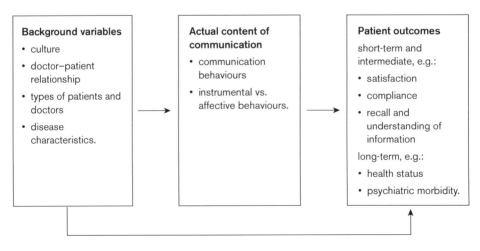

FIGURE 3.1 'Towards a theoretical framework' (Ong *et al.* 1995)

The idea is straightforward. The better we understand, say, 'cultural variables', the better we can specify how they are likely to map on to communication behaviour – and the better we understand that, the better we can specify what the effect will be for patients. Ong *et al.* don't state this, but of course it's clear enough that we cannot specify the communicative behaviour of a particular doctor on a particular occasion, nor how a particular communicative behaviour at a particular moment with a particular patient will affect him or her. However, this doesn't matter, the argument might run. In all epidemiological research we are happy to talk of generalities ('smoking is linked to heart disease') while accepting that the effect on an individual either cannot in principle, or at least cannot at present, be known with certainty.

Thus, broadly speaking, we might have the following:

- *Background variable:* in general, for some cultures, a refusal to make eye contact with someone like a doctor is a mark of respect.
- *Actual content of communication:* the doctor should accept this, and not obtrusively seek eye contact.
- *Patient outcomes:* as a result, the patient will feel more relaxed, more satisfied, and perhaps more willing to enter into partnership with the doctor to address the health problem.

As with all abstract representations, this is too neat to accord with the facts. Here is an authentic example. The doctor is male, in his early thirties, and the patient is a woman in her twenties. My point here is the way that conversation ebbs and flows. Dialogues are process, as is usually said – conversations are constructed. (For transcription conventions, *see* Appendix.)

> Doctor: OK, come in <Fir>. Would you like to come through <Fir>? <silence7> Come and have a seat.
>
> Patient: <inaudible>
>
> Doctor: What can I do for you?
>
> Patient: Erm, well, really it's my hand.
>
> Doctor: Uh huh.
>
> Patient: Cos I've had been having pains in it and it's really swollen/and the vein's really hurting//
>
> Doctor: /right //right
>
> Patient: And then I had pains in my shoulder as well and it sort of spread down my arm.

The patient explains that she has started a new job, working at a bookmaker's:

> Doctor: Right, and that's fairly pressured is it?
>
> Patient: Yeah, yeah, I mean there's races going off every five minutes with people trying to get all their bets off and
>
> Doctor: Right.
>
> Patient: At the last second, so yeah.
>
> Doctor: So you feel under a bit of pressure from that?
>
> Patient: Yeah.

The doctor undertakes a physical examination, which concludes with:

> Doctor: /Right //OK. <PhysS> <phys silence2> Is it tender for me to press anywhere?
>
> Patient: A bit, but not as much as it was.
>
> Doctor: OK.
>
> Patient: It started to get better – I knew it would <laugh>
>
> Doctor: By [zz] of coming to the doctor/ it uh does that on purpose. Can you squeeze my finger? <phys silence> That's OK I think.//
>
> Patient: /<laugh2> //yeh
>
> Doctor: Could you put your hands behind your head? Is your shoulder hurting now?
>
> Patient: It's just a bit tender but <silence>
>
> Doctor: You can't remember straining it or anything/or?
>
> Patient: /No, no
>
> Doctor: Have haven't punched anyone?
>
> Patient: Well, yeah, but was with the other hand.
>
> Doctor: Right. Who did you punch?
>
> Patient: My boyfriend <laugh2>
>
> Doctor: Why was that?

Patient: Well he just annoyed me, so I punched him twice in the face.

Doctor: Is he all right now?

Patient: <laugh> course he is. <PhysF>

The patient asks about blood pressure:

Doctor: Well, I can check your blood pressure if you like it's uh it's/ very unlikely that your blood pressure would give you some sort of swelling and veins in your hand.//

Patient: /<laugh3> //<laugh3>

Doctor: But I'm happy to check it for/you if you'd like.//

Patient: /Oh no //well it's up to you, it's just that I can't think of anything why it's like this, erm my friend was saying that erm it could be something to do with working with [zz]

Doctor: Well it can be, is that uh is there anything repetitive you're doing with your/hand?

Patient: /Yeah, yeah, all the time, on the till, having to do the bets and everything, yeah.

Doctor: And with the till are you pressing with your fingers/ or what?

Patient: /Yeah, yeah, it's mainly with this hand as well.

Doctor: Right. I mean I think your friend is probably right to be honest

Patient: Hmm.

Doctor: It's quite common when you do repetitive movements, it happens to typists/. . .

And the doctor offers a brief explanation of repetitive strain injury and its consequences. He concludes:

Doctor: Well just rest it, ta[ke] are you working over the weekend?

Patient: No, I've got the weekend off now.

Doctor: Take it easy over the weekend, try not to punch your boyfriend/

Patient: /<laugh> That's/ with the other hand, honestly//

Doctor: /and if //if for any reason it swells up again and it's not right then come back and see us, but I think at the moment it may just have been your overusing it on the till, but/ I think it will get better on its own.//

Patient: /yeah //OK. <laugh>

Doctor: All right then? <write5> OK <Fir>, have a good weekend/ then.

Patient: /Thank you, OK. <laugh>

Doctor: Bye for now then.

Patient: Right, thanks a lot.

How would this map on to Ong *et al.*'s framework? First, with regard to 'background variables', one could argue that there is a shared culture here, of sorts. Both participants in the interaction are young, we may assume the doctor is intelligent, and the woman comes across as – at least – bright and alert, whether or not she is educated (during the consultation she mentions that she's going to college, as it happens, as well as doing her new job). The doctor–patient relationship seems relaxed and friendly, perhaps partly for this reason. This manifests itself in certain 'communicative behaviours', particularly in a great deal of laughter during the consultation (it runs all the way through), and in a number of straightforward jokes – again, not all of these are reproduced here. And finally, this seems to have the particular 'patient outcome' of satisfaction with the consultation. This is probably a reasonable interpretation of the fact that the patient's last three utterances include two brief moments of laughter and a concluding, formal 'thanks' which is scaled up to 'thanks a lot.'

The analysis of humour with the apparatus of research inevitably makes the researcher look leaden-footed and humourless. It's a particularly clear instance of a general point, that something as context bound as a dialogue between two people is a fragile, momentary and personal thing, which resists interpretation.

Also, as is often the case, I have had to quote at some length in order to make my point. In other words, the relevant features of the consultation are often hard to identify in the small chunks which a list of skills tends to imply. Rather, they permeate the whole meeting. Indeed, it seems to me that the whole interaction is held together as a successful consultation by such evanescent things as the thread of laughter, the counterpoint between words and physical examination, and so on. To whittle away at these things is to end up with something other than the consultation that takes place. And what advice is there here for the budding doctor? 'Make your patient giggle?' Good idea – and how, exactly?

Thirdly, note that I have set up rules of my own here, and defined the terms of Ong *et al.*'s framework to suit myself – there's nothing to say I can, and nothing to say I can't. This is not a criticism of Ong *et al.* Their framework exists at an entirely abstract level, and they make no effort to flesh it out, but it demonstrates something of the vagueness behind the communication enterprise. The vagueness, I should add, is inevitable in my view. It's just the idea that things aren't vague which is a worry.

However, let's look at things more formally. Does the kind of approach typified by Ong *et al.*, and reported by them, yield information of value?

Evidently, the answer to this question depends on what one means by 'information of value.' As the issues are perceived normally in academic healthcare, there are two stages to this. First, the information must satisfy standards of evidence – it might, for instance, lay claim to statistical significance. If this criterion is fulfilled, then there is the subsequent question of whether it is clinically relevant.

There is, however, a third way of looking at things. Is a particular investigation worth carrying out in the first place? There are two questions here. First, does one research X if the discovery that X is the case is either blindingly obvious or wildly improbable? Can one hope for funds to test the hypothesis that the moon is made of rock, or of green cheese? Secondly, can one hope for funds which have little hope of yielding general conclusions? These might be funds, for example, to discover whether Fred, who used to live in London, has happy memories of his time there, with the results to be disseminated as advice to all doctors: 'Keep off the topic of London with Fred. He didn't like the place.'

In the end, this is a matter for the discourse community to decide. Often, here, the discourse community consists of experts on funding bodies who seek to make judgements about what areas of research to prioritise, and who therefore constantly ask the question 'What is it that we do not know, but which we need to know?' And, as far as individual researchers are concerned, each seeks to build on, extend or disconfirm what has gone before, and in so doing participate in the life and work of the community. Closely related to this, clearly, there is the interactional and persuasive function of science. It takes part in a dialogue designed to do such things as – in a famous phrase – 'create a research space.'[8] That is, one of the things that researchers seek to do is to make a case for a particular area of study being important, under-researched, and therefore potentially theirs. There is also a dialogue which is undertaken to win research grants or journal space in a competitive market, boost one's own career prospects, and so on. The discovery, creation or shaping of knowledge (the metaphor that one chooses reflects different emphases) is in part a matter of saying 'Listen to me – this is how you should look at the world.'

Latour and Woolgar,[4] in a classic study from the 1970s, explore the way in which researchers calibrate and express doubt and certainty in their findings, and what they say is no less relevant in the consideration of how researchers set about choosing what to do. Latour and Woolgar set up five 'statement types' ranging in effect from non-contentious, shared knowledge (Type 5) to 'conjectures' (Type 1). Type 5 statements are 'things that everybody [knows].' They are not mentioned in a paper reporting original research for precisely this reason – their truth may be taken for granted. All rational people agree that the world is round, and that the sun appears each morning to the east. It is not necessary to mention this, nor to reference, say, Columbus and Copernicus in the Bibliography. An explicit statement might seem appropriate, however, in an elementary textbook. Latour and Woolgar label such explicit statements 'Type 4.'

To the researcher, in other words, truth-taken-for-granted has no research value at all. The fact that the sun appears to rise in the east is, in the sense used above, banal. The researcher of today would look naive if an attempt was made to prove it, and the discourse community would not accept it.

Ah yes, one might say, but once upon a time it was necessary to demonstrate such things. Perhaps, but some things are so vastly improbable that research is self-evidently a waste of time, even where we have no direct research evidence – the contrary, in other words, counts as truth-taken-for-granted. I recall reading once of a vicar, in the eighteenth century, who used to advise the ladies in his parish to jump up and down vigorously after what he coyly referred to as 'the marital embrace' as a means of avoiding pregnancy. If this were true, it would revolutionise family planning (and think of the savings to healthcare systems around the world). It is, therefore, an ideal topic for a big research grant – except that it is nonsense. The probable conclusion, 'We found that female post-coital jumping did not affect the probability of pregnancy' states a general truth, but its banality makes it not worth stating.

The moment of counter-intuitive brilliance which leads to something that changes the world happens – but on the whole, what may be assumed need not be researched. Nor, turning to education, need one teach what everybody already takes for granted.

Nor should one teach – turning to Fred, who disliked London – what has little 'surrender value.'[14] This term, borrowed from the insurance business, is used to establish the principle that one teaches what is of frequent utility before one teaches what is of limited utility. For example, a language teacher will teach words with a broad semantic range (e.g. 'laugh', 'cut', 'walk') before teaching those which are more limited (e.g. 'snigger', 'saw', 'hobble').

In other words, research is undertaken in areas where the community agrees it is needed, because the answer to the question cannot be assumed, and may yield results with a surrender value.

Matters of 'truth' and 'fact' (I shall dispense with the prevaricating inverted commas from this point) are of course a lot more contentious than this, as the example of the sun's apparent movement shows. The phrase 'rising sun' is presumably a linguistic hangover from a time when the apparent phenomenon was not known to be illusory – and of course it was with the example of the constancy of the sun's eastern rising that Hume famously challenged the presumptions made based on repeated observation:[15]

> When it is asked, What is the nature of all our reasonings concerning matter of fact? the proper answer seems to be, that they are founded on the relation of cause and effect. When again it is asked, What is the foundation of all our reasonings and conclusions concerning that relation? it may be replied in one word, Experience. But if we still carry on our sifting humor, and ask, What is the foundation of all conclusions from experience? this implies a new question. . . . As to past experience, it can be allowed to give *direct* and *certain* information of those precise objects only, and that precise period of time which fell under its cognizance; But why this experience should be extended to future times and to other objects . . . this is the main question.

Just because the sun has always risen in the east, there is no reason to assume that it will do so tomorrow – although it makes sense to act as if it will. In our terms, therefore, the 'taken for granted' may not necessarily be true. But in the end, however careful we may be as scientists to acknowledge the epistemological status of what we do, we will not get funding for the obvious.

And at this stage we can ask a basic question. Does process-outcome research into clinical communication manage to make statements which are not banal, and not too particular? Is such research, in other words, capable of generalisation beyond the obvious?

Well, the discourse community seems to have an answer to this question. Research is funded, research is published, and the findings are used as evidence. So, to rephrase the question, is the discourse community correct about the area it sketches out between the banal and the idiosyncratic?

Whenever we use language, we make presumptions about what to take for granted. We might, for instance – and for the right reasons – be more likely to reassure a casual work contact that it is nice to see them than a close friend. And, because conventions change from one discourse community to another, different levels of explicitness are required in different contexts. The rules printed on the lid of a board game, say, are not entirely explicit. The rules of

Monopoly do not state that players are not allowed to demand rentals with menaces – this may be understood, even in unusually competitive families. Clinical communication, however – and this is the millstone round its neck – is a discipline which asks for a great deal of explicitness.

The best place to start here is with a paper by Stiles.[16] I quote his Abstract in full:

> A standard criterion for judging the value of a medical interview process component, such as physician information giving, is the degree to which it correlates with positive outcomes, such as patient satisfaction, compliance, or symptom relief. There is a serious problem, however, with this use of correlations. Physicians and patients, like any human beings, give and respond to signals as to what each requires in the interaction. Any such appropriate responsiveness tends to attenuate (and may even reverse) the process-outcome correlation. Under optimum conditions, process components covary with patient requirements but not with outcomes. Thus, for expertly conducted interviews, the expected correlation of process components with outcomes approaches zero, even for components that are causally related to those outcomes.

It is clear what this very formal statement means. The argument is that, because people differ from each other, they will not respond well to the same things. (There is the further point here that, in a world where patients are to be valued and treated as unique individuals, it goes against the grain to treat them as identical.) In other words, the highly proficient doctor will do different things with different people – by extension, his or her communication performance will on particular occasions score relatively poorly against a checklist generated by observation. Note that the point is not that, say, some people are apparently unaffected by a particular communication choice. Some smokers die prematurely, and some do not, but this does not affect the advice that doctors ought to give. The case is worse than that – some people are negatively affected by what is recommended as 'good' communication processes, much as if smoking lowered the risk of lung cancer in certain individuals.

Stiles wanted in this paper to argue against the use of this kind of research. I would want to sustain a weaker version of the same case and say that, given this inevitable variability, the kinds of statements one can make which achieve satisfactory levels of statistical generalisability – they satisfy the conventions of statistics – are at such a level of generality that they are indeed banal. They approach the status of truth taken for granted. They are also, for example, more commonplace than many doctors appreciate. Many of them have been associated with basic teacher-training advice for 30 years or more, for instance.[17]

Or consider the advice offered by Maguire and Pitceathly (cited as reference 19 in Chapter 2) under the heading 'Skills needed to perform key tasks':

> Establish eye contact at the beginning of the consultation and maintain it at reasonable intervals to show interest. Encourage patients to be exact about the sequence in which their problems occurred; ask for dates of key events and about patients' perceptions and feelings . . . Use 'active listening' to clarify what patients are concerned about . . . avoid interrupting before patients have completed important statements.

And so on. All very true, no doubt – but really . . .

To which you may respond: 'Yes, it's true that nothing here is counter-intuitive. But we didn't *know* these things. We merely supposed them – we lacked evidence.' To which the counter-argument is: 'You needed evidence for *this?*'

Consider the contrary case:

> Do not [or, more weakly, 'It is not necessary to . . .'] establish eye contact at the beginning of the consultation, nor maintain it at reasonable intervals to show interest. Do not encourage patients to be exact about the sequence in which their problems occurred; do not ask for dates of key events, nor about patients' perceptions and feelings . . . Do not use 'active listening' to clarify what patients are concerned about . . . interrupt before patients have completed important statements.

Of course, the argument is that without this kind of explicit statement, doctors will not do this kind of thing. This may be so, but that is merely an indictment of the profession, and a very limited justification for the research.

There is a further difficulty, related but not identical. Checklist items retreat into notions of appropriacy (see Maguire and Pitceathly's use of the phrase 'reasonable intervals' above). They do not specify *how much* of a particular skill there should be. Let us agree that some open questions are better than no open questions (I can already hear the reader muttering 'Well, it depends.' Exactly). But are 10 open questions better than 5? Or are 20 better than 10?

The consequences of this are never teased out. Quite simply, we teach certain skills as desirable, we ask students to do them, but there must be some point at which they are doing them too much. After all, if we asked a student to 'confirm patient's understanding' after each phrase, we may presume the consultation would be dysfunctional. And if the response to this objection is 'Well, but the doctor does monitor the patient's understanding to some extent moment by moment, after all. It needn't be a question of explicitly saying "Do you understand?" every five seconds', I would want to respond 'Well, yes – that's exactly my point. Good communication isn't all explicit.' Such unqualified statements as 'confirm patient's understanding' are in fact to be read as meaning 'do this more than you already do.'

The rhetorical nature of the checklist

The main thrust with communication skills research has been in the direction of detail, the identification of particular skills which can be identified, labelled and discussed. The aim in essence has been to put structure on to such amorphous terms as, say, 'bedside manner' by atomising it into its basic behavioural constituents. Checklists therefore include large numbers of micro-skills which, precisely because they are perceptible – they involve sense-data, as the philosophical phrase has it – have the apparent virtue that they can be observed and measured consistently.

How does this work in practice? Suppose we decree that 'Greeting the patient' is a good thing. We might further decree that all and only the following are to be recognised as fulfilling the skill 'greeting the patient': standing up; shaking the patient's hand; smiling; calling them by name. (Why on earth, you might ask, are we to assume that only this is a 'greeting'? But let us leave that for the present.) We now have four marks which can be offered or withheld with a moderate degree of confidence in the reliability of the assessment. If we wish to get really earnest about things, we might decide to specify how perfunctory a handshake needs to be not to count as one, or how prolonged it needs to be to count as embarrassing, and so on. So then let's decide that a handshake has to be of between 1 and 3 seconds' duration. All fine, all measurable. (It may also result in cynical displays of required behaviour by candidates, of course. However, leave that aside too for the moment.)

But what about smiling? Is anyone seriously suggesting that this can be measured objectively? By length? Quality? Teeth? And therein lies the rub. Look once more, for example, at the apparently innocent area of 'eye contact.' We all know that this will vary depending on who we are and who we are talking to. The amount and nature of eye contact certainly vary according to age, culture and sex of the participants, and perhaps in other ways, too. These are Ong *et al.*'s 'background variables.' And they certainly also vary with our own idiosyncratic style of self-presentation, combining with other features of how we appear to the world, creating a persona for ourselves which we are not entirely aware of and perhaps, unless we are very gifted actors, cannot control very much.

In all of these areas, assessment checklists retreat in one of two ways. Either there is use of a poorly defined, pre-theoretically used word or, even more obviously, there is the addition of a prevaricating word which demands subjectivity. Either way, the claims of the checklist are radically reduced. The subjectivity after all allows watchers to award scores that reflect other qualities that they have, such as experience, common sense, wisdom, training, and so on. What value the checklist itself adds, if the researchers do indeed have these qualities, is much less certain, except that it is rhetorically effective. It looks more objective than it is, and the atomisation results in much less than the sum of its constituent parts. Something, that is, has gone missing.

As an example, consider the language of the Maastricht History-taking and Advice Checklist.[18] I want to spend some time on this – although it dates from the late 1980s and a lot of work has been done since then – because it carefully, studiously and honestly addresses the issue of subjectivity head on. That is, the authors understand perfectly well the problems that the methodology creates.

There are two relevant dimensions in the checklist, namely 'interpersonal skills' and 'communicative skills.' The former are broken down into 10 items (numbers 52 to 61), and the latter into 7 items (numbers 62 to 68) (*see* Table 3.1).

Table 3.1 'Interpersonal' and 'communicative' skills from the Maastricht History-taking and Advice Checklist[18]

Interpersonal skills
52. Facilitates the communication
53. Reflects emotions properly
54. Reacts properly to emotions which are directed towards him- or herself as a physician
55. Asks the patient about his or her feelings during the interview
56. Makes, when necessary, meta-communicative statements
57. Performs the history taking and the review of the symptoms properly
58. Puts the patient at ease when necessary
59. Sets the proper pace during the interview
60. Physician's non-verbal behaviour agrees with his or her verbal behaviour
61. Makes proper eye contact with the patient

Communicative skills
62. Uses closed-ended questions properly
63. Concretises at the proper moment
64. Makes proper summaries
65. Provides information in small amounts
66. Checks whether the patient has understood the information
67. When necessary, makes proper confrontations
68. Uses comprehensible language

The instructive thing about this is not so much the particular items which have been selected (some of them are commonplace for this kind of list, and some of them are not), but the points that the authors make in the discussion.

First, they state that 'Reasonable reliability is attained only after substantial training of observers', which indicates – as one would expect – a substantial effort being made to interpret and use the terms on the page. Secondly, for the subscales that we are interested in, it happens that the results are not impressive, as the authors make clear, although they in fact conclude that reliability for 'interpersonal skills' is 'adequate':

> Items in the scale 'interpersonal skills' show low generalisability coefficients (0.00–0.33). Adding a second observer almost doubles the size of the coefficients, although still only low to moderate levels are achieved (0.00–0.50).

> The scale 'communicative skills' displays low levels of inter-observer reliability with the exception of the item on the quality of summaries.

> (0.00–0.29). Increasing the number of observers has very little impact on reliability (0.00–0.44).

However, this is not something that I want to dwell on. There have been studies with less discouraging outcomes. Thirdly, unsurprisingly, the authors point out that:

> High levels of reliability are seen when items are worded in behavioural terms. Low reliability is reported in items that require interpretation by the observers.

Given the range of language offered in the checklist, and the degree of relative subjectivity, this is predictable. It is precisely in clearly defined, objective behaviours that reliability is to be found. If, as we were saying above, we were to award points for the sub-skills involved in 'Greeting the patient', and could define these sub-skills precisely, then anyone could reach the same conclusion about particular performances.

However, there are elements of 'interpretation', at least five different types of which are built into these subscales.

1 Observers were allowed a three-way choice (*yes, indifferent, no*) – quite explicitly as a means of 'allowing a qualitative rating.'
2 There are a range of words all of which mean 'as appropriate.' Thus 'proper/properly' appears 9 times in 17 items, and 'when necessary' appears 3 times.

3   The use of these terms is in itself fairly indiscriminate. For instance, there is no obvious reason why 'Asks the patient about his or her feelings during the interview' is denied the word 'properly.'

4   Words like 'understood' and 'comprehensible' are internally ambiguous. How much 'understanding' is to count as understanding (and how is this to be measured, since it is not easily perceptible)? Does the level of understanding need to be, for example, the same as that of a doctor? Or does it need to be enough for present purposes (and how is this to be defined)?

When it comes to 'comprehensible' the ambiguity is redoubled, because it is unclear whether this is to be interpreted here as 'able to be comprehended' ('What the doctor said was easily comprehensible') or 'actually comprehended' ('What the doctor said was pretty much incomprehensible, but the patient seemed to get the point').

5   And finally there is the word 'small', which is known technically as a 'gradable antonym' – that is, 'smallness' is relative (a small elephant is bigger than a large mouse).

The subjectivity of this part of the checklist is evident, and the authors quite properly insist that the reader is aware of it. It is therefore difficult to see that the list, or these parts of it, achieves anything beyond rhetorical purpose. It has been set out on the page in the same way that an objective instrument is set out, but that does not make it one.

Inevitably, the difficulty is that there have been other such instruments which lack the self-awareness of this one, and where the true function of the checklist is actually to reassure the reader, and beyond the individual reader the discourse community, by offering a clarity and objectivity that are entirely spurious. And, to be clear about this, where such instruments offer advice, we should be aware that such exhortations as 'Maintain appropriate eye contact with the patient' mean 'Look at the patient neither too much nor too little.' This is a game which is not worth the candle.

An alternative position which is quietly set forward from time to time – for example, as part of the SEGUE[19] approach – is to talk in terms of 'frameworks', or some such term, and to keep the actual details of how particular items on a list are manifested deliberately vague:

> For instance, if one task is defined as 'make a personal connection with the patient', students and physicians can proceed in a variety of equally effective ways, choosing one that fits their style, the patient, and the situation. This built-in flexibility with respect to the skills and strategies required to accomplish each task reflects the reality and individuality of human communication. The

> task approach also directs attention toward communication content and process, rather than bedside manner per se.
>
> While it focuses on observable behavior, this approach can facilitate discussion and exploration of attitudes relevant to each task as well.

This is well argued. However, it does overtly break the link between the categories on the list and language, and leaves it to the subjective judgement of the person being assessed what ought to be said, and to the assessor how it ought to be marked, with validation coming from a comparison of raters. There is, I think, little wrong with this as a general approach, however.

What is missing in formal checklists, and what the SEGUE approach lets us glimpse, is a sense of what is known as 'communicative competence' – the difference between the meaning of 'bedside manner' and its constituents, the elusive intuition that makes the difference between the competent and the excellent doctor. The meanings, one might say, between the words – or, more formally, the form-function gap in natural languages.

There are a number of ways of approaching this question, and in the next couple of chapters I shall look at three with which linguists are familiar.

References

1 Gower B. *Scientific Method: an historical and philosophical introduction.* London: Routledge; 1997.
2 Shakespeare W. Troilus and Cressida. In: Wells S, Taylor G, editors. *The Oxford Shakespeare: the complete works* (2e). Oxford: Oxford University Press; 2005 (originally written 1602).
3 Bloor D. *Knowledge and Social Imagery.* London: Routledge and Kegan Paul; 1976.
4 Latour B, Woolgar S. *Laboratory Life: the construction of scientific facts.* Princeton, NJ: Princeton University Press; 1986.
5 Knorr-Cetina K. *Epistemic Cultures: how the sciences make knowledge.* Cambridge, MA: Harvard University Press; 1999.
6 Chalmers A. *Science and its Fabrication.* Buckingham: Open University Press; 1990.
7 Nystrand M. *What Writers Know: the language, process, and structure of written discourse.* New York: Academic Press; 1982.
8 Swales JM. *Genre Analysis: English in academic and research settings.* Cambridge: Cambridge University Press; 1990.
9 Hyland K. Academic attribution: citation and the construction of disciplinary knowledge. *Appl Linguistics.* 1999; **20**: 341–67.
10 Myers G. *Writing Biology: texts in the social construction of scientific knowledge.* Madison, WI: University of Wisconsin Press; 1990.

11 Berkenkotter C, Huckin T. *Genre Knowledge in Disciplinary Communication.* Hillsdale, NJ: Lawrence Erlbaum; 1995.

12 Bazerman C. *Shaping Written Knowledge.* Madison, WI: University of Wisconsin Press; 1989.

13 Horton R. The rhetoric of research. *BMJ.* 1995; **310:** 985–7.

14 Pit Corder S. *Introduction to Applied Linguistics.* Harmondsworth: Penguin; 1973.

15 Hume D (first published in 1748). *An Enquiry Concerning Human Understanding.* Oxford: Clarendon; 2006 (Beauchamp T, editor); www.gutenberg.org/etext/9662 (accessed 12 March 2007).

16 Stiles WB. Evaluating medical interview process components: null correlations with outcomes may be misleading. *Med Care.* 1989; **27:** 212–20.

17 Skelton JR. Everything you were afraid to ask about communication skills. *Br J Gen Pract.* 2005; **55:** 40–46.

18 Kraan H, Crijnen A, Zuidweg J *et al.* Evaluating undergraduate training – a checklist for medical interviewing skills. In: Stewart M, Roter D, editors. *Communicating With Medical Patients.* Newbury Park, CA: Sage; 1989. pp. 167–77.

19 Makoul G. The SEGUE Framework for teaching and assessing communication skills. *Patient Educ Counsel.* 2001; **45:** 23–34.

CHAPTER 4

Two ways of looking at ambiguity

'When I use a word', Humpty Dumpty said in rather a scornful tone, 'it means just what I choose it to mean – neither more nor less.'

'The question is', said Alice, 'whether you can make words mean so many different things.'

'The question is', said Humpty Dumpty, 'which is to be master – that's all' . . .

. . . 'That's a great deal to make one word mean', Alice said in a thoughtful tone.

'When I make a word do a lot of work like that', said Humpty Dumpty, 'I always pay it extra.'

'Oh!' said Alice. She was too much puzzled to make any other remark.

'Ah, you should see 'em come round me of a Saturday night', Humpty Dumpty went on, wagging his head gravely from side to side, 'for to get their wages, you know.'

(Lewis Carroll, *Through the Looking Glass*[1])

Speech Act Theory

One starting point for looking at form, function and ambiguity is what is known as Speech Act Theory. I shall give a little background first, because this has been an extremely productive way of looking at language, but I want in particular to look at the difference between what are known as *locutions, illocutions* and *perlocutions*. (These are not the easiest terms to handle, but you will I hope see that the distinction is straightforward, at least in its essentials.)

We might start with Aristotle, who made a distinction between language used to make statements (which may be regarded as true or false), and the language of rhetoric.[2] This distinction, it has been argued, had 'fateful consequences.' Indeed, '[Aristotle's] remarks ensured that the treatment of non-statement-making sentences came to be banished not merely from logic, but from the realm of science in general.'[3] This is what Aristotle said:

> [N]ot every sentence is a statement-making sentence, but only those in which there is truth or falsity. There is not truth or falsity in all sentences: a prayer is a sentence but is neither true nor false. The present investigation deals with the statement-making sentence; the others we can dismiss, since consideration of them belongs rather to the study of rhetoric or poetry.

The distinction itself is useful. Clearly, not all sentences are true or false. 'Psychiatrists specialise in mental health' is true. 'Most nurses are men' is false. 'Good morning, Jack' is neither.

Aristotle's way of expressing the distinction is echoed, for instance, in contemporary appeals to 'stick to the evidence', to describe fact rather than seek to persuade by rhetorical means. It is the attempt to do so which is, for example, behind the drive for increasingly formulaic, structured research reports in the leading medical journals.[4]

Nevertheless, a point that Smith[3] makes well, Aristotle's way of looking at things covers up a separate point. Language is not merely used to describe, but to make things happen, to have an effect on the world – we seek to *do* things with words. And given in particular that we are concerned with professional language use – where language typically has a professional *purpose* – the idea of categorising language uses in this way is attractive.

It is an understanding that language *does* as well as *describes* that is at the heart of Speech Act Theory. The progenitor of the basic ideas was JL Austin, who died before he could take his proposal very far, but who delivered a series of lectures at Harvard which were subsequently published under the title *How To Do Things With Words*.[5] Austin begins by looking at a class of verbs which he labels *performatives*:

> Utterances can be found . . . such that:
> a. They do not 'describe' or 'report' or constate anything at all, are not 'true or false,' and
> b. The uttering of the sentence is, or is a part of, the doing of an action, which again would not normally be described as, or as 'just', saying something.

This is far from being as paradoxical as it may sound or as I have meanly been trying to make it sound: indeed, the examples now to be given will be disappointing.

Examples:
a. 'I do (sc. take this woman to be my lawful wedded wife)' – as uttered in the course of the marriage ceremony.
b. 'I name this ship the Queen Elizabeth' – as uttered when smashing the bottle against the stern.
c. 'I give and bequeath my watch to my brother' – as occurring in a will.
d. 'I bet you sixpence it will rain tomorrow.'

The point is that in each of these cases, *saying the words* is exactly the same as *doing the action*, provided always that one occupies the correct social role (the bridegroom, the dignitary, and so on). There are many examples of such verbs – for instance, 'I sentence you to five years', 'I declare this fete open', 'You're fired!'

What is particularly interesting from our point of view is the way in which such formal language, as Austin was aware, quickly shows itself to be indistinguishable from the language of everyday use. After all, 'I bet you five pounds they're engaged within the year' (upping the stakes in line with inflation) may well not be intended literally, and may have nothing more than the force of 'I reckon they're pretty serious about each other.' If I say this to you, and I'm wrong, I may very well laugh off your demands for payment in 12 months' time. Similarly, the formal warning that one might encounter in a disciplinary meeting – 'I advise you that giving your identity card to a friend so that he can park on the premises is grounds for disciplinary action' – is echoed less formally in any number of situations. For example, 'A word of warning – do that again and you're in a lot of trouble', 'Take a hint – keep away from my girlfriend', and so on. Until eventually, as Austin was aware, one faces the prospect that everything one says could in principle be preceded by a performative. 'Keep off dairy products' can be prefaced by 'May I suggest that . . .', 'You've got a bit of a bug' can be prefaced by 'I state that . . .', 'How are you today?' can be prefaced by 'I enquire', and so on.

'May I suggest that you keep off dairy products.' As this example shows, explicit performatives often have a formal ring to them. Here, turning from Austin to Austen, are some examples from *Pride and Prejudice*:[6]

> 'So, Lizzy,' said [Mr Bennet] one day, 'your sister is crossed in love, I find. *I congratulate* her. Next to being married, a girl likes to be crossed a little in love now and then.'

Or, from the scene in which Lady Catherine attempts to discover whether the poorly connected Elizabeth seeks to marry Mr Darcy:

> 'This is not to be borne. Miss Bennet, *I insist on* being satisfied. Has he, has my nephew, made you an offer of marriage?'

And finally, here is Lydia Bennet, typically irrepressible:

> 'And in the first place, let us hear what has happened to you all since you went away. Have you seen any pleasant men? Have you had any flirting? I was in great hopes that one of you would have got a husband before you came back. Jane will be quite an old maid soon, *I declare*. She is almost three-and-twenty!'

We do things with words, then. What kind of things?

Austin's untimely death means that the major figure in the development of the theory has been JR Searle. Searle's *Speech Acts*[7] begins with the question 'How do words relate to the world?', and is an extended essay on just this issue. From this, and from subsequent work,[8] I take a few of the basic points.

To answer the question about what kinds of thing we do, he set up five categories:

- **Assertives:** these are statements about what we perceive the world to be. In making an assertive, we are describing the world as we perceive it to be.
- **Commissives:** these commit the speaker to a course of action. They are associated with verbs of promising, offering, etc. With commissives, we commit ourselves to altering the world as it is.
- **Directives:** these are typically orders, requests and the like. With directives, we commit someone else to changing the world as it is. (The concept of changing the state of things as they are by issuing a directive is neatly captured in the *Star Trek* command: 'Make it so.')

In addition to these central uses of language, Searle proposes two other categories:

- **Expressives:** these describe the psychological state of the speaker. We pass comment on how, for instance, the assertives that we utter make us feel.

And, finally:

- **Declaratives:** these are in essence performatives – verbs which, if uttered by the right person, bring into being the state of affairs that they describe.

So, for example, we might have:

- **Assertive:** That Rottweiler of yours *is* very large, Peter.
- **Commissive:** Sheila and I *can* take him for a walk if you want.
- **Directive:** Damn thing bit me. *Could* you just pass me its muzzle, Sheila dearest?
- **Expressive:** *I'm glad* I'm a police officer.
- **Declarative:** Peter, I *arrest* you for failing to control a dangerous animal.

By this account, everything one says can be reduced to the following:

- This is how things are.
- I'll change how things are.
- Please change how things are.

Then, in addition to this, there are the special cases of declaratives, where doing and saying collide, and of expressives, where the state of the world is related to the psychological state of the speaker. It is through expressives, in other words, that we are able to stand back from the world and comment upon it.

In one sense, performatives (or declaratives) look simply like a linguistic curiosity, but there is more to them than that. As Searle observed, they fulfil the God-like role of language, captured by the author of Genesis:

> In the beginning was the word . . .
> . . . God said, 'Let there be light, and there was light.'

The promulgation of laws is also an obvious place to look for performatives in action – consider the common UK legal phrase 'A new offence has been created.' And artists, and for that matter teachers of art, too, show us new ways of looking at the world. They show us 'ways of seeing', in Berger's phrase.[9] Or, as Wallace Stevens said, writing (or so it is often suggested) about Picasso's much-reproduced Blue period 'The old guitarist':

> They said, 'You have a blue guitar
> You do not play things as they are.'
>
> The man replied, 'Things as they are
> Are changed upon the blue guitar.'[10]

Among other things, therefore, what is at stake here is the way in which we use language to shape the world we live in, and which – subject as we are to the human condition – we are obliged to try to make sense of.

Why Speech Act Theory matters

What I'm trying to do here is to break language open for the reader, to give a sense of how it operates, and of what the relationship between the speaker and the world is like. In addition, there are I think two important points, which are concerned not with the philosophy of language, but with the psychology of language in action.

The first point is that patients have a dangerous habit of taking doctors seriously. This means that what doctors tell patients about themselves, about their conditions, and about their prognoses, tends to assume the status of a truth. Doctors, in other words, create ways of seeing for their patients – when they state that something is the case, they make it so.

This may not matter. After all, the world is full of facts. If a patient is told 'You have asthma', and the doctor is competent, there is a weight of evidence to support the statement. However, there are plenty of areas where the evidence is less certain, or where guidelines change, or where labels are offered that might be withheld – for example, 'Your blood pressure is too high', 'You're drinking too much', or even 'You're not very well.' Truth and illness can be medical creations.

With regard to the central trio, of assertives, commissives and directives, we have a summary of a great deal of purposive interaction. If we are doing things with words, buying a train ticket or talking to a patient, it is through these three speech act types that we achieve our goals. There is an underlying pattern in consultations, for instance, which runs:

> Patient: I declare that I suffer.
>
> Doctor: I commit myself to assisting you.
> I direct you to take your medication.

Or, of course, in a patient-centred, concordant world:

> Patient: I declare that I suffer.
>
> Doctor: I commit myself to assisting you.
> We will decide on your medication together.

In the latter example, the rights of committing and directing are both mutually shared.

This underlying structure resembles what I have argued for elsewhere, in a study of pronoun and verb use in primary care.[11] There is an emerging pattern here, we proposed, of:

Patient: I suffer.

Doctor: I reflect.
We act.

These are abstract, deep patterns (I don't imply intellectual profundity on my part, but merely that these patterns are far removed from the surface of text – from the words that are actually spoken), and for that reason they are extremely simple. They are, nevertheless, worth bearing in mind.

Ambiguity and narrative: locution, illocution and perlocution

There is one central consideration, however, which brings us to the next stage in the argument, and that is, as we have seen, that language does not necessarily mean in use what we think it might mean. Not all utterances which look like assertives actually function as assertives. For example, an apparent declarative ('I bet you five pounds', as above) may not be literally meant, and so on.

To solve this problem, Austin suggested a three-way distinction into what he called *locution, illocution* and *perlocution*. This distinction has been much discussed, modified and reinterpreted since, initially and most notably by Searle. I should stress that there are different ways of looking at the distinction, that the arguments they involve are much more subtle than I am implying here, and that my account is a simplification. However, for our purposes we might say that, roughly speaking, *locution* is apparent, propositional meaning, *illocution* is concerned with the intention of the speaker, and *perlocution* is concerned with the effect on the listener (the phrases 'illocutionary force' and 'perlocutionary effect' are often used).[12]

Why is this relevant? Part of the ambiguity of language in use is that the same phrases may differ with regard to locution, illocution and perlocution. For example, the phrase 'It's hot in here', which is propositional (it might reasonably elicit a true/false reply – 'Yes, you're right'), might have the illocutionary force of a request – 'Do you mind opening the window?' However, it might have the effect of causing an insult.

We may imagine a very eminent professor and a young research assistant. When he murmurs 'It's hot in here', she may reply 'I take it, Professor, you're not suggesting I slip into something more comfortable? Is this the kind of thing you say to all your assistants?' (You will note in passing that the phrase 'Why don't you slip into something more comfortable?' has, conventionally, the perlocutionary effect of 'Why don't you change into sexually provocative clothes?', rather than 'Put on your dressing gown and slippers, dear, while I make you a nice cup of cocoa.')

What matters in particular is the difference between *intention* and *effect*. Sometimes we play on this ambiguity quite deliberately – the language of seduction being, in fact, a pretty good example. Let us suppose, for instance, that our professor is foolish enough to believe that the aphrodisiac effect of his eminence is sufficient to outweigh the disadvantages of middle age, paunch, pomposity and a wife *in situ*. Perhaps he really does hope that his assistant will at once demurely unbutton. However, when she reveals the quiet contempt in which he is in fact held ('Don't be ridiculous!'), he has his response ready: 'My dear young lady, I was merely complaining about the heat!' Or, if they are both linguists with a pedantic turn of mind: 'My dear young lady, the illocutionary intent of what I said was merely to *complain*, not to *persuade* you to do something so evidently alien to your nature and contrary to good professional relations. Or, in strictly speech act terms, what you took to be a Directive was a simple, harmless Assertive. Now, would you be a good girl, make me a cup of tea, and we'll forget all about it.'

Ambiguity between intention and effect can be used for creative purposes as well. As a teenager, I was neatly tricked in Paris by a youth who was presumably making a political point. He walked up to me on the street and asked '*Vous avez un franc?*', and when I replied '*Non*', he gave me one.

Or, more seriously, there is the background to the decision to use the atom bomb on Japan:

> In his press conference of July 27 1945, [Japanese] Prime Minister Suzuki Kantaro, responding to the terms of the Potsdam Declaration [which demanded the surrender of the Japanese] said that the government's attitude was one of *mokusatsu suru*. This was taken by the Allies to mean 'treat with silent contempt' and a rejection of their terms, when in fact the *Mainichi Daily News* has [subsequently] argued that Suzuki's **intended** meaning was 'no comment.' . . . According to the *Mainichi* the government had in fact already decided to accept the Potsdam Declaration. The result of this confusion was the prolongation of the war and the atomic bombing of two Japanese cities.[13]

However, as President Truman later recalled it, 'They told me to go to hell, words to that **effect**'[14] (my emphasis in both cases).

In one sense, this draws attention both to the role of language and to the importance of the intention/effect distinction. At the same time, however, a word of warning is needed. If one looks hard enough, and defines that voracious term 'communication' broadly enough, and allows weak enough links between causes and effects to be recognised, then most accidents, misfortunes and mishaps can be repackaged as 'communication problems.' Johnson's point above, for example, is what he dryly describes as the 'tendency of the Japanese [in political life] to take refuge in alleged mistranslations' rather than to make the case for a breakdown in communication. The frequency with which 'communication' is cited in complaints against doctors (*see* Chapter 2) needs to be seen with this cautionary note.

Ambiguity pervades what we do, and is central to our ability to manage our relationships with other people, to protect ourselves and negotiate our way through the day without causing offence. At times, it is built in and formulaic (e.g. 'Do you want to come to the cinema with me?', 'I'm washing my hair'). Or consider the elaborate language of the widely used 'Pendleton's Rules' – for example when a doctor has attempted a role-play session in front of a group of peers. The procedure can be roughly summarised as follows.
1 Briefly clarify matters of fact.
2 The doctor speaks first and describes/discusses 'what went well.'
3 The rest of the group then describe/discuss 'what went well.'
4 The doctor describes/discusses 'what could have been done differently.'
5 The rest of the group then describe/discuss 'what could have been done differently.'

This is a way of formalising feedback, and ensuring that no one is at risk of having their performance torn to pieces by a critical audience. However, it is clear that the illocutionary force of 'What could have been done differently?' is 'What went badly?' Undergraduate medical students are good at healthy cynicism and routinely accustomed to criticism from teachers. They have as a consequence a slight tendency to laughter if they are invited to use 'done differently' rather than 'went badly', particularly where their own performance is concerned. They recognise the game for what it is. Qualified doctors, with more professional pride at stake, can occasionally be grateful for the shield of courtesy.

This is a kind of creative, more or less deliberate ambiguity. It is seen in a very different and more serious context in discussions of serious illness, where it centres on words like 'stable.'[15] There is a gap here between ordinary language use and technical language use. Ordinary language use suggests a meaning that is something like 'unchanging.' Technical language use seems to mean something like 'not having changed for some time, and not likely to change in the immediate future' – an ambiguity that is neatly demonstrated by the phrase 'He's stable for the moment.'

This, in ordinary language terms, is getting into the area of white lies and respecting other people's feelings.

> 'How does this dress make me look?' asked Mrs Smith.
>
> Her husband glanced up from the newspaper. 'Mutton dressed as lamb', he said.

I expect they're divorced by now. Words don't weigh the same. This is not a situation that is redeemable by a single compliment. You can't counteract the use of a single racist term, say, by a single apology ('Oh, sorry, it sort of slipped out'). In recent times a football commentator in the UK, thinking that his microphone was switched off, expressed exasperation by describing one of the players in racist terms. His remark destroyed his media career. You can't boost a colleague's morale, or motivate a class, by telling them once they're doing well for each time you tell them they're doing badly.

And so it is that we have:

> 'How does this dress make me look?' asked Mrs Smith.
>
> Her husband glanced up from the newspaper. 'Mutton dressed as lamb', he thought to himself anxiously.
>
> 'Well', he said slowly. 'I'm not sure it's really you. I mean, you have such a lovely figure after all . . . What about that blue one – you look great in that.'

Ambiguity, prevarication, politeness, respect for others – however you want to label it, we talk in riddles a great deal of the time. Uncertainty is at the heart of language, and our ability to disambiguate partly but not wholly, and not always to look too closely at ways of disambiguating which might hurt us, is at the heart of our ability to make some limited sense of our world and the people we meet.

The fact is that consultations are complex, because a great deal of communication is complex. The fact is also that there are many ways to analyse a consultation, but that the essence of the task is to preserve the ambiguity of what happens from time to time, and more to the point to preserve the fact that communication is not so much ambivalent through and through, but multivalent. Speakers do many things at the same time. Here, using just the apparatus discussed in this chapter, is a fairly routine example, which shows the decision-making component of the consultation.

An elderly woman is here accompanied by her husband. The husband has recently been in hospital, and has also bought a car. The woman has a number of problems she wants to mention. One is her ankle, which the doctor has just examined (for transcription conventions, *see* Appendix):

> Doctor: It's a nasty bruise you've got there, isn't it – how did you get that?

The first part of this utterance does three things. First, it is an Assertive – it states what is the case. And, as the speaker is a doctor, and therefore giving an expert view, it has something of the 'God-like role' of language of which Searle speaks. It is, in other words, a kind of Performative – 'I declare your bruise to be nasty.' And therefore, of course, the doctor is saying that the patient and her companion are justified in bringing the issue to his professional attention. And, of course, it is also an Expressive – the doctor is offering an expression of sympathy, indicated by the invitation to the patient to agree ('isn't it?'). The Assertive therefore has the illocutionary intention of both reassurance and sympathy.

> C: /yes she's removed the flesh, she did this to her to her ankle or erm six months/ ago it took weeks and weeks to heal/ up
>
> Doctor: /yes /they take ages to go don't they. Oh it's not too bad sorry. OK right well you've got a little wound there you're going to need that covered up for erm quite a few days I think.

Again the doctor uses a tag question ('don't they') to indicate agreement. There is then a further Assertive ('you're going to need . . .' etc.), which is apparently intended as a Directive (it's a piece of advice as to how the state of affairs should change). The advice is softened by the phrase 'I think', which is an Expressive, of sorts, which may be designed to soften either the whole sentence, or just the recommended length of time, or both.

> Patient: yes/
>
> C: /hmm.
>
> Doctor: Let's/ cover it up.

The use of 'let's', the second piece of doctor language which might look like a local piece of 'shared decision making', functions as both a Directive and a Commissive – that is, it appears to be both an offer and a request.

There has been a brief earlier discussion about the new car. The patient now, a little ruefully, remarks that she has recently had a birthday:

> Doctor: Did he buy you a nice present?
>
> C: I couldn't I was/ <inaudible> well I was back but I couldn't get out you you've/ had three presents dear, yes she's had three presents.
>
> Doctor: /oh you were in hospital.

> Patient: /<inaudible> I'm glad you mentioned it.
>
> Doctor: He probably bought that car to share with you I expect.
>
> Patient: <laugh> I expect <laugh>.
>
> C: I've got mine shortly too.
>
> Doctor: So is it bright red this new car?
>
> C: Yeah oh bright red yes/
>
> Doctor: /Had to be I could just see you in nothing else but a bright red car.
>
> Patient: <laugh>

The consultation drifts in and out of this kind of gentle, personalised banter. The purpose – all consultations are best regarded as purposive – is to consolidate the relationship, and to consolidate trust. Therefore, given that there is in fact an apparently high degree of trust already present, the rules about how the doctor can successfully advise change. In other words, just as we are often less formal with those we know and trust (we don't need to offer the elaborate structures of politeness as a defence), so advice can be offered with less effort to develop a shared decision:

> Doctor: Brilliant OK now what are we going to do about that arm, are you going to let nurse have a look at it again in a few days/ time?
>
> C: /yeh yes please yes please.

(Notice in passing a UK commonplace – the professional label 'nurse' used without an article, as if it was a proper name, like 'Mary.') The perlocutionary effect of the interrogative is that an offer is being made (i.e. it's a Commissive – and it isn't a question). The response ('yes please yes please') seems to make this clear.

> Doctor: I would have thought that that dressing's fine but I would have thought you ought just to let her have a look at it in the middle of next week/ to make sure that it's/

Of course, '. . . you ought to' etc. is advice giving. It is softened by the repeated Expressive 'I would have thought . . .' Altogether, between this brief quotation and the next few lines of text, advice is given seven times, but never explicitly negotiated. Not all the advice giving is reproduced here, in the interests of space.

Clearly, without a fairly subjective view of what constitutes 'shared decision making', we are going to say there is none present here.

Eventually the consultation draws to an end. I've reproduced the leave-taking element in full, because it is protracted, friendly and indicates how successful the consultation has been:

> Doctor: Don't lose your scarf/ come and see nurse erm book it now come and see nurse sort of middle of next week and just/ let her check that arm that it's going on all right.
>
> Patient: /No.
>
> Companion: /All right thank you very much doctor.
>
> Doctor: And erm I hope you stay well.
>
> Companion: Uh huh.
>
> Patient: Thank you very much/
>
> Doctor: /I'll see you again, nice to see you, bye bye.
>
> Patient: Bye bye.
>
> Doctor: Bye.
>
> Patient: Have you stick stick oh it's there.
>
> Doctor: Don't look as though you need a stick.
>
> Companion: Yes I visit erm <name of hospital> first Thursday of next month.
>
> Doctor: Good all right hope all goes well for you.
>
> Companion: Cheers.
>
> Patient: Thank you very much.
>
> Doctor: Bye bye/ now bye.
>
> Companion: /Bye doctor thank you very much.
>
> Doctor: Bye.

And here, as has happened throughout, a lot of things are happening at the same time.

I have used this consultation as an example of how familiarity changes the rules of use – or rather, how familiarity of the particular type and to the particular extent of just these people on just this occasion have changed them, so that what is clearly a friendly and supportive meeting fails to represent a great many of the standard communication skills prerequisites, particularly around sharing decisions.

This returns us, by a different route, to the question of the banal and the particular which I spoke of as being parameters in what to research. We can say that these words work on this occasion, but the surrender value is slight. What is *particular* about this is what makes it successful. But beyond the usual vacuous generalisations (the patient is listened to and so on), there is little to say of general worth. Such is language. If the relationship between words and meanings was arbitrary, we could not communicate. If it was an absolutely precise fit, it is hard to see what the point of both language and number would be.

This is among the topics that Swift satirises, as Gulliver visits a fictitious place of learning, the Academy of Lagado.[16] This, too, is a search for certainty in a world of uncertain meaning:

> [T]hree professors sat in consultation . . .
>
> . . . An expedient was . . . offered, 'that since words are only names for things, it would be more convenient for all men to carry about them such things as were necessary to express a particular business they are to discourse on.'
>
> And this invention would certainly have taken place, to the great ease as well as health of the subject, if the women, in conjunction with the vulgar and illiterate, had not threatened to raise a rebellion unless they might be allowed the liberty to speak with their tongues, after the manner of their forefathers; such constant irreconcilable enemies to science are the common people . . .
>
> . . . Another great advantage proposed by this invention was that it would serve as a universal language, to be understood in all civilised nations, whose goods and utensils are generally of the same kind, or nearly resembling, so that their uses might easily be comprehended.

In this light, the call for structured discussions in journal papers, which seems just like irritated common sense, might perhaps begin to look like a chase after an ignis fatuus, a dream of academic objectivity.

Communicative competence

If there are potential ambiguities all the time in language, how do we manage to understand each other at all? What process-outcome research tends to demonstrate, by showing that it cannot entirely predict cause and effect, is that there is another quality which is itself not amenable to rule, certainly not at present and probably not in principle.

I used the phrase 'rules of use' a few moments ago. Languages are indeed rule governed, but they are not completely rule governed. English has 'grammar rules', for example – such as 'except in the case of a finite and well-defined list of verbs, you form the past tense by adding {ed} to the verb stem thus: "watch"/"watched."' This is known as a 'rule of usage.' However, it tells you nothing about when to use the past tense – in writing up the Results section in a research paper, for example, as I found to my cost. Similarly, part of the discourse of some sports seems to be for players to use what is commonly known as the 'historic present' for the sake of vividness, when a past tense might seem temporally more appropriate – for example, 'So Giggsy crosses to me and I gets me head to it and there it is in the back of the net.' And a common way of making a tentative, formal request is to begin with a past tense where actually the time reference is present – for example, 'I wanted to ask you if I could possibly have a couple of days off work . . .' Here the past tense seems to function as a marker of professional inferiority.

These 'rules' ('for some sports, sportsmen can use the historic present') are known as 'rules of use', and although we all know many of these intuitively in our own language, no one has ever tried to specify what the complete set of 'rules of use' are, not least because the rules change all the time, and from place to place. Think about how word meanings change, and who can use these words, and when, over a generation. The word 'gay' is a frequently mentioned example. Although it seems very occasionally to have been used to mean 'homosexual' from the 1930s,[17] this is not acknowledged in standard dictionaries through the 1980s and beyond. Yet now the earlier range of meanings has been entirely supplanted.

How large, pervasive and problematical a phenomenon this is, however, is best illustrated by unfamiliar languages, where the unfamiliarity brings home to us how much we take for granted in our own language. This is Dell Hymes, looking at the way questions are handled in different 'speech communities.' He is talking about the way that children acquire, without realising it, the kind of understanding which allows them to apply 'rules of use' correctly:

> From a finite experience of speech acts and their interdependence with sociocultural features, [children] develop a general theory of the speaking appropriate in their community . . . e.g. among the Araucanians of Chile, that to repeat a question is to insult; among the Tzeltal of Chiapas, Mexico, that a direct question is not properly asked (and to be answered 'nothing'); among the Cahinahua of Brazil, that a direct answer to a first question implies that the

answerer has no time to talk, a vague answer that the question will be answered directly the second time . . .

This is from Hymes' classic paper (it is beautifully written, although this is a rather clumsy sentence, you may think), entitled 'On communicative competence',[18] which is the first detailed statement of this concept. I don't at this stage propose to go into the theoretical underpinning of this exhaustively discussed topic, except to pick up a famous phrase from Hymes:

> There are rules of use without which the rules of grammar would be useless.

The fact is that the micro-skills of clinical communication are, in essence, attempts to capture rules of use by indicating the effect that a piece of language will have on a hearer ('in order to have effect X, say Y'). That is, they are attempts to specify what the relevant pieces of communicative competence are, or what the link is between illocutionary intent and perlocutionary effect.

However, this can only be done in a rough and ready way. Those who are non-native speakers of a language, for example, will still get things a little wrong from time to time, however good they are. A Japanese student once said to me, of what I would have called a T-shirt, '*That's a nice top you're wearing, John.*' Possibly a successful compliment to a woman, but not quite right (or would you disagree?) for a man. The semantic range of possible uses of a word like 'top' is a tiny, localised example of communicative competence, as are the rules of use (you might like to introspect about these for a few minutes or, if you are not a native speaker, consider how hard it is to do so with confidence) governing who could say them. The Japanese student was female, for example, so is her comment therefore 'more appropriate' than it would have been from a man?

A natural language contains vast numbers of rules of use, most of which, probably, have not been explicitly recognised, but all of which we know if we have native-speaker intuition, and are at home with the context of utterance – that is, with the cultural, social (and professional) context in which we are speaking. For example, I might define myself as British, middle-class, Caucasian . . . and so on. Within this context I communicate with a degree of confidence. At work I try to monitor myself, as we all do, and develop an understanding, say, of when to make jokes, and when not to, of whether I can use first names, of how to stay within the 'real me', as I conceive myself to be, presenting to the world a professionalised accommodation with my private self, and so on. The extent to which I do this well or badly contributes to people's view of me as a good or poor communicator. And if I seriously lack this nuanced understanding even in my home culture, then perhaps my clinical colleagues will begin to worry that I am on the autistic spectrum.

On the other hand, I visit other cultures professionally quite often. Under these circumstances, my communicative competence is less – sometimes much reduced, in fact – and two things happen. First, I present a much more neutral version of myself, to reduce the risk of appearing foolish or insulting. I will therefore inevitably appear in a less idiosyncratic, less personalised light, and generally present myself as a more formal (and very possibly duller) individual. Then, secondly, I rely on the goodwill of my hosts to recognise that I'm in unfamiliar territory, and that I'm at least trying.

The point is that the question of how to use language to present oneself in a certain way – or to create effects with listeners – is exceptionally difficult. We cannot specify all the rules of use, and finer and finer explorations of what they are is pointless, at least if the aim is to arrive at a set of instructions about how to behave.

WB Yeats wrote this poem,[19] a piece of passionate declamation which concludes with lines that many will recognise:

> Never shall a young man,
> Thrown into despair
> By those great honey-coloured
> Ramparts at your ear,
> Love you for yourself alone
> And not your yellow hair.
>
> But I can get a hair-dye
> And set such colour there,
> Brown, or black, or carrot,
> That young men in despair
> May love me for myself alone
> And not my yellow hair.
>
> I heard an old religious man
> But yesternight declare
> That he had found a text to prove
> That only God, my dear,
> Could love you for yourself alone
> And not your yellow hair.

The lady's hair is described as 'yellow', a word which is very common in the language and, although one not normally associated with poetry perhaps, a word which works perfectly in context. Poets, particularly relatively modern ones such as Yeats, have often felt themselves to be under pressure to use unusual words, more particularising words. So why should one not offer something more particular here? Indeed, given the link already in the poem between hair and foodstuffs ('honey-coloured/ramparts'), what about, maybe, 'corn-coloured'? That would work, but unfortunately it doesn't scan. So what about 'custard', then? That would fit the rhythm:

> . . . only God, my dear,
> Could love you for yourself alone
> And not your custard hair.

Perhaps not. But why? Well, just because. This isn't the kind of connotation that custard has in English – or carrot, hence the lady's dismissive reference to 'carrot'-coloured hair dye. (These things are culture-specific. The original words for Chinese foodstuffs normally translated into English as 'dumplings' have none of the connotations of risibility that, somehow, the word 'dumpling' has.)

However, the implications have to do with many more things than culture. The question of what is odd, and whether it gets accepted in context, is far more complicated (and the ostensibly weird is far more common) than one is aware of, either at the time or later. Here are a GP and a patient in consultation. The latter has just finished explaining her symptoms (for transcription conventions, *see* Appendix):

> Patient: What would that be?
>
> Doctor: Well, it's probably your arthritis isn't it? I mean at your age you're going to have a little bit of arthritis in your back.
>
> Patient: I know I've got arthritis. I can't lie on my head at night. It's as if –
>
> Doctor: On your head?
>
> Patient: Yeah. I've had that for years. It's as if I'm lying on {zz}
>
> Doctor: Right.
>
> Patient: I have to keep manoeuvring about till I find exhausted find a place and fall asleep.

Notice how far we are here from the world of either the checklist or the more generalised accounts of what happens in consultations. But this is authentic, and – from the tape – it appears that both parties took it in their stride.

One final point here – what is a question, exactly? Consider:

- So you're going at two o'clock?
- How do you do?
- Have you got the price of a cup of tea?
- Do you want a good hiding?

. . . or what about 'an inquisitive glance'? I've put a question mark after each of these phrases, but for no particular reason. We could easily claim that the first, said with the appropriate intonation, is a confirmation, that the second is purely formulaic, that the third is a request and that the fourth is a warning to behave better.

None of this is exactly new – this kind of issue is basic to linguistic enquiry. There is a distinction to be made between the formal, grammatical category of 'Interrogative', easily identified because the verb inverts ('have you got?' as opposed to 'you've got') or, as above, because a 'tag' ('isn't it') is added, or an auxiliary is put in place ('do you have?') – and the functional category of 'Question', which needn't be grammatically marked. The result is that not all Interrogatives are Questions, or vice versa.

Nor, in general, can language forms be mapped on to language functions, or vice versa. There are typical patterns, typical ways of fulfilling the function of 'making a request', and so on. These are often grouped together in language textbooks, which have frequently been functionally organised since the 1970s. From this it will be clear that we don't really *know* objectively what constitutes the function 'asking a question' (we can't use an ordinary grammar as the sole evidence for it), which means that we must interpret such terms subjectively. As it happens, we can do so fairly successfully, because we have communicative competence. However, we should not pretend that this is an exact science, or that we are likely to understand all the functions of a conversation that is undertaken by two other people.

Vygotsky, in one of the most evocative and profound reflections on language ever written,[20] makes exactly this point in a discussion of, among other things, acting – actors, of course, being masters of the art of extracting all sorts of different meanings from the same series of words. He quotes Dostoevsky's *Diary of a Writer*:

> One Sunday night I happened to walk for some fifteen paces next to a group of six drunken young workmen, and I suddenly realised that all thoughts, feelings and even a whole chain of reasoning could be expressed by that one noun, which is moreover extremely short. One young fellow said it harshly and forcefully, to express his utter contempt for whatever it was they had all been talking

about. Another answered with the same noun but in a quite different tone and sense – doubting that the negative attitude of the first one was warranted. A third suddenly became incensed against the first and roughly intruded on the conversation, excitedly shouting the same noun, this time as a curse and obscenity. Here the second fellow interfered again, angry at the third, the aggressor, and restraining him, in the sense of 'Now why do you have to butt in, we were discussing things quietly and here you come and start swearing.' And he told this whole thought in one word, the same venerable word, except that he also raised his hand and put it on the third fellow's shoulder. All at once a fourth, the youngest of the group, who had kept silent till then, probably having suddenly found a solution to the original difficulty which had started the argument, raised his hand in a transport of joy and shouted . . . Eureka, do you think? I have it? No, not eureka and not I have it; he repeated the same unprintable noun, one word, merely one word, but with ecstasy, in a shriek of delight – which was apparently too strong, because the sixth and the oldest, a glum-looking fellow, did not like it and cut the infantile joy of the other one short, addressing him in a sullen, exhortative bass and repeating . . . yes, still the same noun, forbidden in the presence of ladies but which this time clearly meant 'What are you yelling yourself hoarse for?' So, without uttering a single other word, they repeated that one beloved word six times in a row, one after another, and understood one another completely.

It could almost be an exercise in an actor's workshop.

References

1 Carroll L. *Alice's Adventures in Wonderland and Through the Looking-Glass.* Harmondsworth: Penguin; 2004 (first published 1871).
2 Ross WD (written *c.*350BC) (Edghill EM, trans.). *The Works of Aristotle. Volume 1. Categoriae and De Interpretatione.* London: Oxford University Press; 1928; http://classics.mit.edu/Aristotle/interpretation.html (accessed 13 March 2007).
3 Smith B. An essay on material necessity. In: Hanson P, Hunter B, editors. Return of the A Priori. *Can J Philosophy.* 1992; **Suppl. 18:** 301–22.
4 Docherty M, Smith R. The case for structuring the discussion of scientific papers. *BMJ.* 1999; **318:** 1224–5.
5 Austin JL. *How To Do Things With Words.* Oxford: Clarendon Press; 1962.
6 Austen J (first published 1813) (Kinsley J, editor). *Pride and Prejudice.* Oxford: Oxford University Press; 2004.
7 Searle JR. *Speech Acts: an essay in the philosophy of language.* Cambridge: Cambridge University Press; 1969.
8 Searle JR. A taxonomy of illocutionary acts. In: Gunderson K, editor. *Language, Mind and Knowledge.* Minneapolis, MN: University of Minnesota Press; 1975.

pp. 344–69. (Also in Searle JR. *Expression and Meaning: studies in the theory of speech acts.* Cambridge: Cambridge University Press; 1979. pp. 1–19.)

9 Berger J (first published 1973). *Ways of Seeing.* Harmondsworth: Penguin; 1990 (reprint edition).

10 Stevens W. The man with the blue guitar. In: *Collected Poems.* London: Faber and Faber; 2006 (first published in Stevens W. *The Man with the Blue Guitar*, 1937).

11 Skelton JR, Wearn AM, Hobbs FDR. 'I' and 'we': a concordance analysis of how doctors and patients use first-person pronouns in primary care consultations. *Fam Pract.* 2002; **19**: 484–8.

12 Lyons J. *Semantics. Volumes 1 and 2.* Cambridge: Cambridge University Press; 1977.

13 Johnson C. Omote (explicit) and ura (implicit): translating Japanese political terms. *J Japanese Stud.* 1980; **6**: 89–115.

14 Ferrell RH. *Truman and the Bomb: a documentary history.* Worland, WY: High Plains Publishing Co.; 1996.

15 Skelton JR, Murray J, Hobbs FDR. Imprecision in medical communication: an exploratory concordance and protocol study of a doctor talking to patients with serious illness. *J R Soc Med.* 1999; **92**: 620–5.

16 Swift J. *Gulliver's Travels.* Harmondsworth: Penguin; 1994 (first published in 1726 as *Travels into Several Remote Nations of the World*).

17 Harper D. *On-line Etymology Dictionary*; http://dictionary.reference.com/browse/gay (accessed 5 April 2007).

18 Hymes D. On communicative competence. In: Pride JB, Holmes J, editors. *Sociolinguistics: selected readings.* Harmondsworth: Penguin; 1972. pp. 269–93.

19 Yeats WB. For Anne Gregory. In: Finneran RJ, editor. *Collected Works of WB Yeats: the Poems.* London: Prentice Hall and IBD; 1997 (first published in 1933 in *The Winding Stair and Other Poems*).

20 Vygotsky LS. *Thought and Language.* New York: MIT Press and John Wiley & Sons; 1962.

CHAPTER 5

An old debate

... Raphael, though descended from eight uninterrupted genera-
tions of painters, had to learn to paint apparently as if no Anzio
had ever handled a brush before. But he had also to learn to
breathe, and digest, and circulate his blood ... he had to begin
as a speck of protoplasm, and to struggle through an embryonic
lifetime, during part of which he was indistinguishable from an
embryonic dog, and had neither a skull nor a backbone ... He
had to compress untold centuries of development into nine months
before he was human enough to break loose as an independent
being. And even then he was still so incomplete that his parents
might well have exclaimed, 'Good heavens! Have you learnt
nothing from our experience that you come into the world in
this ridiculously elementary state? Why can't you talk and walk
and paint and behave decently?' To that question baby Raphael
had no answer.

(JB Lamarck, *Zoological Philosophy*[1])

Introduction

In this chapter I focus on the still extant but now rather elderly debate between
'behaviourism' and 'mentalism', as represented respectively by Skinner and
Chomsky. Secondly, I want to look at the concept of 'patient-centredness',
beginning with the sophisticated analysis by Mead and Bowers,[2] one of a series
of important papers that they undertook around this topic. Thirdly, I want to
touch briefly on the role of qualitative research in the discourse community,

and the view of the relationship between language and thought embedded in it.

More on causes and effects

The great comedian Marty Feldman had a comic routine in which he set out to test the hypothesis that the use of certain language could 'corrupt and deprave' (this being the legal phrase associated with the UK law on pornography). Feldman played the human guinea pig in an experiment, sitting in a laboratory and confronted by a scientist (with white coat and clipboard) and, between the two, a pretty young woman. The scientist gravely read off a list of potentially corrupting phrases from the list on the clipboard, each perfectly enunciated and followed by slow, careful scrutiny of the research subject. 'Firm young thighs' was perhaps one of the phrases. As the test sentences became more extreme – although all in fact were fairly tame – Feldman grew increasingly agitated until at last, duly corrupted by the power of words alone, he flung himself on the woman.

This is funny because we know that this is not how language works. Yet 'Science', as Thomas Hobbes said,[3] 'is the knowledge of consequences and the dependence of facts upon one another.' The point is that communication does not have this kind of immediate dependence. Feldman is not – and we are not – guinea pigs.

The study of cause and effect works best when the self-awareness of the subject cannot intervene – and relatively poorly, we may imagine, when the object of enquiry is language, precisely that resource which allows people to define and demonstrate their self-awareness, and to modify what they say and think. Languages themselves are subject to change through time and place, sometimes quickly, sometimes slowly, but either way inexorably, as individuals make choices about language use and language fashion. You are polite, or abrupt, or angry, or affectionate in a way that is different from me, and both of us are so in a manner that is different to our parents, and so on – until over the centuries we have to read our ancestors in translation.

This is one reason why the whittling down of communication can feel so crass. It runs counter to what we think ourselves to be. There is a certain irony in this. Communication skills are a standard-bearer for the contemporary, humanistic and holistic view of what medicine should be. Yet we have asked the scientist to take it seriously by looking at it with narrowly scientific methodologies. The result is often mechanistic. At extremes, this leaves us with this kind of thing being explored as a possibility at the University of Florida:[4]

> We are exploring using virtual characters to help educate patient–doctor communication skills. Our current system allows medical students to interview DIANA, a virtual patient. Students interact with DIANA naturally using speech and gestures. A virtual instructor, VIC, provides immediate feedback on the student's performance.

DIANA is indeed a representation of a young woman (she is wearing, for some reason, a kind of leotard, and her legs are implausibly long). Students interact with her, and among other things '[h]ead tracking data shows where the medical student is looking during the interview', so that they may therefore look at an image of DIANA with green spots superimposed to indicate where their gaze has been. The idea is that with 'immersion' in this kind of simulation, students will develop their skills.

This approach, let it at once be conceded, is vulnerable, and it is unfair to leave the methodology to stand or fall on its own without reference to how it is used. For present purposes the real virtue in drawing attention to it is to demonstrate the logical conclusion of a retreat into scientific measurement.

This is all really an argument about the status of observable behaviour. No one could deny that, in seeking to understand other people, what we have to go on is what they do and what we make of it. In other words, we have to start with perception. What is at stake is the extent to which we can take the perceptible at face value (specifying some piece of behaviour as being predictably 'good' in its consequences, or as representing some state of the mind). In other words, it's a question of how much we allow ourselves to interpret.

And, as you will have observed, I used the word 'mind', which was originally what this kind of psychological approach was designed to get away from.

This takes us to the heart of two competing traditions, usually summed up as 'mentalist' versus 'behaviourist.' I take up some aspects of this issue here, but make no claims to an exhaustive summary. Pinker has provided an excellent recent discussion,[5] and for an up-to-date, thorough and clear version of the issues surrounding behaviourism and language, the reader is referred to Owen.[6]

In the early years of the twentieth century, psychologists began to recognise how amorphous, open-ended and subjective their terminology was. This was one of the driving forces behind behaviourism, and I should perhaps pause to mention very briefly a few of the names that are typically cited as relevant here.

One of the central aims of behaviourism was to rigorously use precise terms for phenomena which were observable pieces of behaviour – and by extension to eliminate from enquiry what was not observable, and therefore what had to be considered unscientific. In his classic manifesto, Watson[7] says:

> Psychology as the behaviourist views it is a purely objective experimental branch
> of natural sciences . . . Introspection forms no essential part of its methods, nor
> is the scientific value of its data dependent upon the readiness with which they
> lend themselves to interpretation in terms of consciousness.

The roots of the discipline, by common consent, lie partly in the philosophical
tradition of Associations, particularly as developed by Hume – although Hume's
scepticism about the relationship between cause and effect was as far from
behaviourist theory as it is possible to get. Hume's view was that experiences
have nothing substantial underpinning them, that (as we saw earlier) the link
between cause and consequence is one we assume, and that therefore we make
sense of the world by noting common associations – of cause and effect, of
resemblance, and of continuity. John Locke is another name usually mentioned
in this context,[8] principally because he was the most influential proponent of
the idea of the *tabula rasa* – the view that when we are born our minds are 'blank
tablets' on which experience writes. This, logically enough, led him to a belief
in the importance of education:[9]

> I think I may say that of all the men we meet with, nine parts of ten are what
> they are, good or evil, useful or not, by their education.

Locke's belief in education was also a belief in helping people to think, and
to reflect on their state and the world around them – which is where he and
behaviourism as applied to educational theory differ.

Partly also the roots of behaviourism lie in logical positivism,[10] which sought
to analyse apparently nebulous, non-empirical concepts such as 'beliefs' not in
terms of an individual having a state of mind, but in terms of their propensity to
behave in certain ways under certain circumstances. A belief in God, according
to this view, is not best described in terms of a list of accompanying beliefs,
or of a certain general attitude towards one's fellow creatures, or to creation.
Rather, it is represented by such things as a predisposition to pray at certain
points, to fast according to set routines, and so on. And of course there is the
kind of experimental work that was pioneered by Pavlov,[11] involving the study
of stimulus–response behaviour in animals – in Pavlov's case, famously, in dogs.
Here is one of the key moments in his work, as Pavlov described it. He writes, as
you will observe, with great clarity and precision:

> . . . as no special stimulus is applied the salivary glands remain quite inactive. But
> when the sounds from a beating metronome are allowed to fall upon the ear, a
> salivary secretion begins after 9 seconds, and in the course of 45 seconds eleven

drops have been secreted. The activity of the salivary gland has thus been called into play by impulses of sound – a stimulus quite alien to food. This activity of the salivary gland cannot be regarded as anything else than a component of the alimentary reflex. Besides the secretory, the motor component of the food reflex is also very apparent in experiments of this kind. In this very experiment the dog turns in the direction from which it has been customary to present the food and begins to lick its lips vigorously.

Animals can be trained in certain ways, and can by constant repetition of tasks and by reinforcement on successful completion (giving them a morsel of food, for example) be trained to push buttons, to run mazes and the like. This is what learning is. The world is a mechanical place. There are stimuli. We respond to them. Our habits are reinforced when we receive gratification as a consequence. There is a push-button relationship between cause and effect or, as some people phrase it, a 'billiard ball' relationship. However, as this analogy is Hume's, and as he introduced it for different purposes, I shall stick to the former metaphor.

The consequences are well illustrated by that area of education where behaviourist learning caught on, namely the teaching of languages. In particular, in the USA, the advent of war in 1941 brought with it an urgent need to learn the languages of friend and foe alike. What developed as a methodology during the war and afterwards was largely based on stimulus–response theory.[12] It was first called 'Army Method', but later this transmuted into the Audio-Lingual Method (or ALM), and the latter is a more familiar phrase. (This way of putting it probably makes the whole initiative seem more coherent than it actually was. For some fascinating background, see Roger Dingman's account of the experiences of the US Marine Corps language instructors learning, and later using, Japanese as part of the war effort.[13])

The end of ALM is no less interesting. In a massive educational research project, students were exposed to either ALM or 'traditional' teaching. The results were fairly devastating, to the point of being, as the lead researcher acknowledged, 'personally traumatic to the project staff.'[14] ALM as a methodology performed less well, and to all intents and purposes disappeared, at least as a thoroughgoing account of 'good method.'

At any rate the fundamental idea of behaviourist teaching was, as with the 'teaching' of rats, a matter of *stimulus*, *response* and *reinforcement*:

Stimulus: What's this?

Response: It's a book.

Reinforcement: Good.

Unadulterated behaviourism of any kind, in fact, seldom happens in teaching today, but it remains common practice as a way of giving beginner language teachers (and teachers in general) a lesson in an unfamiliar language, to show them what it's like to learn something apparently from zero, and to help them introspect about how they learn. Here, keeping with the theme of Japanese, is a slightly tidied up transcript of a lesson taught to a group of health professionals seeking to develop as teachers:

T:	Kore wa, nan desu ka?	*What's this?*
	Kore wa nan desu ka?	*What's this?*
	Hon desu.	*It's a book.*
	Hon desu. (Pause 2)	*It's a book. (Pause 2)*
	Kore wa, nan desu ka?	*What's this?*
	Hon desu. (Pause 2)	*It's a book (Pause 2)*
	Kore wa, nan desu ka?	*What's this?*
S1:	Hon desu	*It's a book.*
T:	Hai. Hon desu. Hon desu.	*Yes. It's a book. It's a book.*
	Kore wa, nan desu ka?	*What's this?*
S2:	Hon desu	*It's a book.*
T:	Hai.	*Yes.*
	Kore wa, nan desu ka?	*What's this?*
S3:	Hon desu.	*It's a book.*
	Hai, hon desu. Hon desu.	*Yes, it's a book. It's a book.*

Setting a transcript out in the cold light of day like this is a way, really, of emphasising some of the problems of the methodology – the lack of application to any real-world use, the mind-numbing boredom of the approach (a commonly used term of approbation for the endless cycles of repetition was 'overteaching'), and a general air of manipulative barrenness. Yet to an extent this is unfair. The level of challenge for the complete beginner is very considerable (these totally unfamiliar words, the sounds never heard before, and the inevitable failure to get to grips with the grammatical constituents of a language so distant from English), and the tension in the classroom – for better or worse – can as a consequence be high. In short bursts boredom, strangely, is the last thing on anybody's mind – the students are too busy trying to keep up.

Behaviourism as an intellectual discipline, represented here by the endless slog of overteaching as good habits are inculcated, bad habits suppressed (positively and negatively reinforced, in the language of the trade), has in its rigour a whiff of Calvinistic self-denial. These days, as Pinker[5] points out, 'Strict behaviourism is pretty much dead in psychology, but many of its attitudes live on' (p. 21). To which one might add, in all fairness, that the approach certainly has its point, which one might reasonably sum up as follows – science not waffle, observation not hunches.

Radical behaviourism, to give this branch of the movement its more descriptive title, is most commonly associated with the name of Skinner, who among other things over a long and productive career, wrote explicitly about communication – or, as he called it in the title of his book, *Verbal Behaviour*.[15] When the book was published, Skinner was already in his fifties, although as it turned out he still had many active years before him, and to an extent it was seen as a culmination of many aspects of his thinking. And it was almost immediately demolished in a review[16] by Noam Chomsky, at that time a young man, just turned 30, but with one discipline-changing book already under his belt, who went on to become certainly the most influential linguist of his generation, and perhaps the most influential of all time. (He has also had a substantial influence on education, although he has not necessarily welcomed it. And in recent years a version of some of his ideas has reappeared in neuro-linguistic programming.[17])

The review is an extraordinary tour de force, vigorous and confident, and displays all the fierce rhetorical brilliance that Chomsky has demonstrated throughout his career (perhaps to compensate for his formal work in linguistics, which is staggeringly technical, and unreadable for those who haven't been through a long period of initiation). Indeed, Chomsky is so much the exemplar of the researcher as rhetorician that this particular aspect of his work has itself been studied by linguists and political commentators – not all of them well disposed to a man who for many years now has been a leading spokesperson for the American Left.[18,19]

One of his central points in this review is to note that Skinner's apparent precision in his use of terms is spurious – the attempt at a kind of purging of the language of psychology simply fails. This is Chomsky on stimulus and response:

> We can, in the face of presently available evidence, continue to maintain the lawfulness of the relation between stimulus and response only by depriving them of their objective character. A typical example of *stimulus control* for Skinner

would be the response to a piece of music with the utterance *Mozart* or to a painting with the response *Dutch*. These responses are asserted to be 'under the control of extremely subtle properties' of the physical object or event. Suppose instead of saying *Dutch* we had said *Clashes with the wallpaper, I thought you liked abstract work, Never saw it before, Tilted, Hanging too low, Beautiful, Hideous, Remember our camping trip last summer?*, or whatever else might come into our minds when looking at a picture . . . Skinner could only say that each of these responses is under the control of some other stimulus property of the physical object. If we look at a red chair and say *red*, the response is under the control of the stimulus *redness*; if we say *chair*, it is under the control of the collection of properties . . . *chairness* (110), and similarly for any other response. This device is as simple as it is empty. Since properties are free for the asking . . . we can account for a wide class of responses in terms of Skinnerian functional analysis by identifying the *controlling stimuli*. But the word *stimulus* has lost all objectivity in this usage. Stimuli are no longer part of the outside physical world; they are driven back into the organism.

And he concludes by reiterating the same point:

The terms borrowed from experimental psychology simply lose their objective meaning with this extension, and take over the full vagueness of ordinary language.

This, of course, carries a distant echo of the ostensible precision of the language of checklists. However, Chomsky's mental dexterity is such that paraphrasing him can be risky, a point brilliantly caught in Botha's exhilarating survey of the main arguments for and against his work over the years.[20] But in his own words, written for a brief Preface published alongside a reprint of the original some years later:[16]

I had intended this review not specifically as a criticism of Skinner's speculations regarding language, but rather as a more general critique of behaviorist (I would now prefer to say 'empiricist') speculation as to the nature of higher mental processes. My reason for discussing Skinner's book in such detail was that it was the most careful and thoroughgoing presentation of such speculations, an evaluation that I feel is still accurate. Therefore, if the conclusions I attempted to substantiate in the review are correct, as I believe they are, then Skinner's work can be regarded as, in effect, a *reductio ad absurdum* of behaviorist assumptions. My personal view is that it is a definite merit, not a defect, of Skinner's work that it can be used for this purpose, and it was for this reason that I tried to deal with it fairly exhaustively . . . I do not . . . see any way in which his proposals can be substantially improved within the general framework of behaviorist or neobehaviorist, or, more generally, empiricist ideas that has dominated much of modern linguistics, psychology, and philosophy. The conclusion that I hoped to establish in the review, by discussing these speculations in their most explicit and detailed form, was that the general point of view was largely mythology, and that its widespread acceptance is not the result of empirical support, persuasive reasoning, or the absence of a plausible alternative.

That is to say, he believes that we learn language not primarily as a result of the environment around us, and the way that it reinforces particular patterns of behaviour, but as a result of heredity. We have what he called a 'Language Acquisition Device' in the brain. It is this question of heredity which Lamarck sets out in his light-hearted discussion of Raphael above. Some things we inherit, some things we learn – some things, that is, are already written on what is therefore not quite the *tabula rasa* we are born with.

A simple formulation of this aspect of Chomsky comes in the following interview from 1983 with the psychologist and journalist John Gliedman – and published, a little improbably, in the science fiction magazine *Omni*:[21]

> Question: Why do you believe that language behavior critically depends on the existence of a genetically preprogrammed language organ in the brain?
>
> Chomsky: There's a lot of linguistic evidence to support this contention. But even in advance of detailed linguistic research, we should expect heredity to play a major role in language because there is really no other way to account for the fact that children learn to speak in the first place.
>
> Question: What do you mean?
>
> Chomsky: Consider something that everybody agrees is due to heredity – the fact that humans develop arms rather than wings. Why do we believe this? Well, since nothing in the fetal environments of the human or bird embryo can account for the differences between birds and men, we assume that heredity must be responsible. In fact, if someone came along and said that a bird embryo is somehow 'trained' to grow wings, people would just laugh, even though embryologists lack anything like a detailed understanding of how genes regulate embryological development.

It's the environment that accounts for the fact that a child learns Italian rather than Swahili, say, but the fact that we recognise language at all, that we come to use it, that we understand its purposes, that we recognise the relationship between the word and the world and so on – these go unremarked (basic coursebooks in Italian don't say 'Italians use words to talk to each other') because we take them for granted. 'It is precisely what seems self-evident', Chomsky remarks, 'that is most likely to be part of our hereditary baggage.'

This is one of the great research conundrums. How do you explore what cannot be directly perceived, such as the things of the mind? Do you act as if the imperceptible does not exist, at least for the purposes of scientific enquiry?

It also hints at one of the great questions of human knowledge, mockingly known since Ryle's criticism of Cartesian dualism[22] as the question of whether there is a 'ghost in the machine', whether there are things in human behaviour that cannot be explained in terms of the operations of human bodies (as opposed to 'minds'). Ryle, a positivist, argued that there were not. However, this is a debate that I don't intend to enter more deeply. From the educationalist's point of view, what matters, I would want to argue, is this:

For our purposes, there are three different ways in which the word 'imperceptible' might be used, and we should be careful about what we mean. For example, in ordinary language use, we might say that the movement of a glacier is 'imperceptibly slow', but this of course does not mean that glaciers do not move, nor that this movement is in principle impossible to measure. Merely, it is not usually perceived. But in fact, using only the relatively poor instrument which is our sight, the movement of the glacier, the opening of a flower, a sunset – any slow thing – can be seen if we glance at it (that is, take occasional sample measurements) from time to time. From the gathering darkness now and the hint of twilight half an hour ago, we fill in the intermediate stages and deduce the continuous process. Secondly, we might say that certain sub-atomic particles have never been directly observed, but that their existence can be hypothesised as a result of certain other effects which have been directly observed. The observed movements (substitute, for humans, observed behaviours) act as a proxy measure for the existence of the object – or quality, for humans – we are interested in. And thirdly, when we describe something as 'imperceptible', we may simply mean that we are not conscious of noticing things which in fact we have noticed. And a great deal of communication is like this – it is part of the definition of communication that it can be perceived, but part of life that we often don't notice it consciously.

As educators, therefore, we must face the fact that it is often difficult to measure or describe aspects of communication, and some of these aspects in any case are ephemeral. Therefore we must decide to what extent we can treat sense data, or behaviour, which we notice as a proxy for such things as attitudes, values or competence. As I have tried to stress, I believe that attitudes and values are best treated as educationally real, and as motivating behaviour rather than merely being the sum of all the behaviours.

The question is therefore whether we can get successfully from behaviour to value. How much (to pick up a phrase from the paper by Mead and Bower[2] considered below) is 'lost in translation'?

The great patient-centred conundrum

Here is an apparent example of 'patient-centredness' in action from the GP database (for transcription conventions, *see* Appendix). The patient has just been told by her GP that she has genital warts. The fact that these are sexually transmitted is handled with tact, with the doctor – also female – concluding:

> Doctor: [the infection happened] a while ago probably they they could be infectious at the moment so your present partner could get them.
>
> Patient: OK.
>
> Doctor: OK any other questions?
>
> Patient: Erm not really.
>
> Doctor: Clearish?
>
> Patient: But I was just about to start going on the pill <laugh>
>
> Doctor: Erm no no that's fine that's fine but but yeah I mean do you want to use condoms with the pill that's the only question I mean it is safer against
>
> Patient: Well I mean if you if you suggest using condoms then obviously I should erm but shall I bother starting the pill till this is all sort of cleared up type th[ing]?
>
> Doctor: Well that's up to you the that's what I was just saying th[e] th[e] the only advantage of that or the main advantage is that should the condom split or anything or something go wrong then you have got that protection.
>
> Patient: Yeah.

How can we defend this as 'patient-centred'? Well, we might draw attention to what I have called the doctor's 'tact' throughout the discussion, which can be evidenced through the written text only by quoting at great length (from an audio version one would pick up the tone of voice). This is fairly subjective either way. Then there is the explanation which immediately precedes the segment quoted, which in turn leads to an invitation for questions, which – as often happens – the patient does not take up. The doctor persists ('Clearish?'), and the patient, offered the opportunity a second time to take things further, does so. She was considering going on the pill, which raises the issue of the use of condoms while she's infected. This is presented as a clear choice for the patient – 'it's up to you.'

Well, that's all very patient-centred, but we should explore this in detail. First, there's the use of the question 'I mean do you want to use condoms with the pill . . .?' and secondly the phrase 'it's up to you.'

These are precisely the kinds of things that are taken as objective evidence of a patient-centred approach. One is a question used to establish an attitude of mind rather than to elicit clinical information. The other is an explicit invitation to act as the decision maker.

Yet of course the invitation is less real than that – its illocutionary intent is more difficult to get at. We may suppose that if the patient had declined to use condoms, the doctor's response would probably not be 'OK then.' From this we might conclude that, unless the doctor was really prepared to let the patient endanger the health of her partner, the offer of patient-centredness is not real.

'It's up to you', for instance, can mean a number of different things. Change the intonation, and you have in effect:

> It's up to you (whether you want to behave like a completely irresponsible idiot).

Or alternatively:

> It's up to you (frankly, I can't be bothered).

Or, as Mead and Bower expressed it in their classic overview of patient-centredness,[2] one of a number of studies undertaken by this team, 'non-specific verbal behaviours have no inherent relation to higher-order concepts such as "sharing power and responsibility."'

One aspect of this problem can be most neatly put as a familiar conundrum. If the doctor offers a patient-centred (negotiating, mutualistic, etc.) consultation, and the patient says 'I leave it up to you, doc', is it then patient-centred to do what the patient asks and behave in a doctor-centred manner? Is it patient-centred to be doctor-centred?

And then again, there is still more to our example than that. The fact is that on tape the two key phrases come and go in a low-key way. It's easy to interpret them as markers of politeness rather than anything else – the question asked in the full expectation that the answer to the question, and the final choice, will be the clinically appropriate one. In other words, the doctor is *doing* patient-centredness, but she isn't *being* patient-centred in the sense of offering genuine choice. Her intention, in other words, may actually be no more than 'observe my patient-centredness.' She is perhaps creating an undercurrent of patient-centredness which may not be real, as would be clear if the patient took her up on the offer (if the patient's perlocutionary uptake was that an offer had been made), but which is part of the overall style of the doctor and conduct of the consultation.

And beyond that, there is the possibility that the doctor is not entirely attentive at this moment, and makes a routine comment out of habit.

This is a question of whether 'patient-centredness' is best considered as a set of gestures (a combination of setting, language, paralanguage, and so on), or a state of mind. Whether, in other words, it is on the surface, a set of behaviours to enact, or underneath. If we define it as the latter, if it is indeed sometimes possible to be patient-centred in attitude by being doctor-centred in manner, then we are talking about a need to understand people's intentions. This must mean using as our resources either a set of tools – checklists of behaviour – which are a poor fit for the job (see Mead and Bower's comment above, and Stiles, cited in Chapter 3, page 52), or a subjectivity which at best we can dress up as insight and common sense, but which is not a research tool at all, as normally considered.

'Insight' and 'common sense' are also vague terms, as indeed are many of those surrounding 'patient-centredness.'

Mead and Bower suggest five dimensions.[2]

1 **Biopsychosocial perspective.** 'Many illnesses', they point out, '. . . cannot adequately be assigned to conventional disease taxonomies.' 'Illness' and 'disease' are not co-terminous. 'Broadening the explanatory perspective on illness to include social and psychological factors has expanded the remit of medicine into the realm of ostensibly "healthy" bodies.'

2 **The 'patient as person.'** Everyone is different. '[I]n order to understand illness and alleviate suffering, medicine must first understand the personal meaning of illness for the patient.'

3 **Sharing power and responsibility.** Referring back to Byrne and Long's seminal study of 1976,[23] the authors state that 'the theme of sharing medical power is an almost universal element of published descriptions [of patient-centredness] since then.'

4 **The therapeutic alliance.** This is 'a fundamental requirement rather than a useful addition.' It includes Rogers' 'core therapist attitudes of empathy, congruence and unconditional positive regard.'

5 **The 'doctor-as-person.'** This concerns 'the influence of the personal qualities of the doctor.' Balint *et al.*[24] are cited: 'the doctor and patient are influencing each other all the time and cannot be considered separately.'

All of these dimensions except the last one, the authors suggest, have been studied, with varying degrees of success. The fact that the last dimension has *not* been studied, they argue, 'reflect[s] the difficulty of operationalising such a complex and content-specific variable.'

However, this is not intended to be a complete list – the dimensions are generalising labels to sum up aspects of the research that has been conducted. No particular claim is made that they cover all and only the aspects of patient-centredness, nor that the labels themselves are mutually exclusive. Indeed, as the authors point out, all of them interact with each other. They merge fairly effortlessly into one, and out again to several every time one looks at them. Could we not, for instance, subsume the concept of the 'patient as person' under the psychosocial part of the triaxial consultation which is dimension 1? Or could we not, on the contrary, argue that there are other dimensions to be *added* to the triaxial consultation, not normally considered under this heading, but not considered – or not clearly considered – elsewhere in Mead and Bower's analysis?

For example, just as every consultation will have a psychosocial element which may sometimes be trivial and sometimes be central, so every consultation will have an ethical element, which may or may not be in the foreground. Every consultation will also have an interactional element – doctor and patient will need to establish and sustain some form of ordinary human relationship, governed by our social understanding of the kind of thing we may say, and the kind of way we may act, under these circumstances.

This suggests that, rather than the triaxial consultation developed in the early 1970s,[25] we might work with a 'pentaxial consultation' – although it is difficult to talk in this free-and-easy way about adjusting models so soon after quoting Chomsky's criticism of 'properties [which] are free for the asking.' (Why not a 'spiritual' dimension, too? And you may be able to think of others.) Thus we might have the following elements, one or more of which will be in the foreground of the consultation:

- biological
- psychological
- social
- ethical
- interactional.

The 'interactional' aspect is best illustrated when things go wrong. We developed a scenario many years ago – to be honest for a little light relief – of a young woman who is meeting her doctor for the first time. The role player involved is under instructions to try to arrange a social meeting with the doctor, as a date if it's a man, and on a 'let's be best friends' basis if it's a woman. There are a number of interesting things about the scenario. First, it offers to perfection examples of the differences in illocutionary intention and perlocutionary uptake – the scenario typically consists of a series of polite refusals from the doctor, which are not interpreted correctly by the patient. Secondly, the patient inevitably comes across as lonely and unhappy, because she clearly has problems generally with making sense of the interactional world – it's difficult to imagine her having many friends, for example. Her communicative competence is poor. Thirdly, medical students in particular, as opposed to qualified doctors, tend to play the game by the wrong rules. They offer polite excuses which the patient, precisely because the social game confuses her, doesn't notice as such. So you get this kind of thing:

> Doctor: No, I couldn't possibly meet you this evening – we work very late at the practice, and I'm tired by the end of the day . . .

> Patient: Well, what about at the weekend then? We could meet on Saturday, perhaps? There's a good film on . . .

And so on. What is needed is a clear statement – 'I can't meet you this evening because you're my patient.' The rules of the language game at this stage are professional, not social, and if the norms of politeness are not understood by one party then this point must be made in other ways. Politeness proceeds by indirection, but only so much indirection as is compatible with getting the message across. And indeed it also becomes clear, when this scenario is attempted, that the doctor cannot help this particular patient until the interactional side of things is sorted out.

If you want, you can incorporate these terms elsewhere. 'Interaction' might come under 'therapeutic relationship', or the 'social' element of 'biopsychosocial' – 'spirituality', you might say, is part of the 'psychology' element – why not? However, this is pointless juggling and, in the case of spirituality, a good example of how presuppositions are built into one's understanding of centredness. We may suppose that an atheist and a believer will disagree about whether spirituality can be roughly bundled up as a subset of something else in this way. All of these terms – including the ones I have just added – are inherently imprecise. They also have something which is a classic feature of language, namely meaning shaped by context.

As the authors point out, the central difficulty is that 'the proposed conceptual framework does not map neatly on to some of the measures reviewed.' And, a little later, 'It is a common fact that complex theoretical concepts cannot be adequately translated into practical measures, but it is important to be clear about what is lost in translation.' Precisely. To put it less theoretically, where patient-centredness is concerned, how do you know that power has been shared?

Let me put this as strongly as possible. 'Patient-centredness' is poorly defined. No one seems quite sure whether it exists as a yearning (an imperceptible, unscientific yearning) inside the head of the doctor or the patient, whether it is a set of things to do or things to think, or a compendium of things to say. I suspect, in fact, that its use is so wide, that it is so invariably a term used for approbation, that it means little more than 'good.' In this context, let us ask the following blunt question. Does patient-centredness exist?

As I write this, I am of course overcome by a need to reassure the reader that I, too, believe in good things – but in a way that's exactly my point.

Qualitative research

There are areas where quantitative study can give you nothing *except* numbers. It doesn't follow, however, that qualitative research can provide an answer, or at least, that it can provide an answer to the question 'How do we do successful communication with patients?'

The limitations of research are facts of life, whether the kind of research being done is the most mechanically frequentative or the most gushingly subjective. Nothing ever really tells us what the case is. This hardly matters, provided always that we know how ham-fisted our efforts are – and have the resilience to plough on, refining and refining if necessary until we have inched a little closer to how things are.

However, the true value of qualitative research is what it can offer under certain circumstances. Quantitative research can give us what, conventionally, we accept as evidence on matters which are susceptible to quantitative study. 'Which is superior – treatment x or treatment y?' is the archetype of this kind of enquiry. Qualitative research claims to give us something which, by a different set of conventions, we accept as evidence. It is therefore best used on matters which, although not susceptible to quantitative enquiry, we nevertheless need an answer to. Clearly there are many such things in academic medicine. The problem of professionalism is a case in point, as we have seen. Communication is another.

I want to concentrate on some of the issues here by looking at Mishler's classic qualitative study of doctor–patient interaction,[26] dating from 1984. This is partly simply because it is good in itself, but principally because it demonstrates neatly the irreducibility of qualitative research, and therefore mirrors the irreducibility of many of those issues which engage us in communication-based research. It is not, as it happens, featured among the studies reviewed by Ong *et al.*, nor incidentally by the Toronto statement, even though the latter study concludes by remarking that 'Qualitative methods need to be encouraged.' These are telling omissions.

Mishler's central point is sometimes summed up as a distinction between the 'voice of medicine' and the 'voice of the lifeworld', with the former being associated with the doctor and the latter with the patient, although as Mishler points out, the notion of 'voice' stems from Silverman and Torode.[27] However, Mishler's discussion is more than this conveniently memorable contrast makes it seem. He argues first of all that:

> Physicians' control of structure is matched by their control of content. The relevance and appropriateness of information is defined through what physicians choose to attend and ask about. This bounded domain of relevance is summarized as the voice of medicine. Occasionally the flow of the interview is interrupted by the 'voice of the lifeworld' when patients refer to the personal and social contexts of their problems. Physicians rapidly repair such disruptions and reassert the voice of medicine.

This way of putting it seemed perhaps more novel when it was written than it does now – doctors these days at least know that they are supposed to be aware of the personal and social context. But in any case Mishler declares himself (*see* Chapter 3) dissatisfied with this analysis. It says too little about social theory – a problem which Mishler identifies in much of the literature on doctor–patient interaction up to that date – and one might add that this is a problem that has persisted:

> Reports tend to be limited to presentations of empirical findings or to narrowly focused interpretations that neither place such interviews in broader contexts nor relate them to more general theoretical issues.

He then sets out to reanalyse his findings, drawing on two traditions in social theory. The first of these is that of Schutz,[28] who distinguished different 'provinces of meaning.' One of these provinces, which is shared by all, is the 'natural' attitude – the world is as it appears to be. We can only negotiate it in our daily lives by accepting it at face value. ('The world of working in daily life is the archetype of our experience of reality. All the other provinces of meaning may be considered as its modifications', according to Schutz.) Yet doctors, for example, are trained to develop a 'scientific' attitude, one in which the subjective immersion in the process of living is replaced by an objective, 'disinterested' mindset. (The word 'disinterested' here – satisfying for the semantic purist – means 'neutral', not 'lacking in interest.') And there is, argues Mishler, a 'fairly close congruence' between Schutz's distinction and his own.

This line of argument is clear enough, and there is enough truth in it to make it worth considering, but it is also a little unfair. Good 'scientific' doctors (those who understand the points that David Bloor was making 30 years ago) are well enough aware of the relativistic arguments, and well enough aware of the extent to which science 'provides answers' rather than, say, explanations which fit the data and have pragmatic value. It seems unfair to look at those who no doubt do subscribe somewhat unthinkingly to a naive scientism, and oppose to them the many who are more profound thinkers on the other side of the fence. As Noordhof expresses it very neatly:[29]

> 'Scientism' is a term of abuse . . . A successful accusation of scientism usually relies upon a restrictive conception of the sciences and an optimistic conception of the arts as hitherto practised. Nobody espouses scientism; it is just detected in the writings of others.

However, for the moment we will let Schutz's broad distinction go unchallenged – we may presume, after all, that the doctor who did not attempt a degree of objectivity was not doing his or her duty. And certainly, if we were ill, we would none of us be pleased by a doctor who was as disabled by our fears and anxieties as we were ourselves. In the end – a point that is sometimes overlooked in the general rush to patient-centred empathy – objective application of specialist expertise is what we want and what we pay for, after all.

Habermas,[30] turning to Mishler's other social theorist, distinguishes between 'symbolic interaction', which is essentially interaction designed to foster and strengthen social norms, and 'purposive–rational' interaction, which is essentially concerned with the language of the workplace. And this language is itself less concerned with social norms beyond the workplace, and more with getting things done. There is a risk, Habermas argues, that 'the institutional framework of society' will be '*absorbed* by the subsystems of purposive–rational interaction.' It is this point which Mishler picks up:

> I am proposing that the dominance of the voice of medicine is an example of the 'absorption' of ordinary language by the system of purposive–rational

action. In analyses of medical interviews, undertaken from the patient's point of view, I have shown that this leads to an 'objectification' of the patient, to a stripping away of the lifeworld contexts of patient problems. For this reason I have concluded that such a form of discourse severely limits, if it does not exclude entirely, the possibility of humane medical practice.

This, then, is Mishler's central argument. Rephrased in the kind of language that is more familiar in academic medicine, the doctor's agenda and health beliefs dominate the structure and content of the consultation, and the fact that they do so is an instance of an overarching principle in action – the goal-oriented language of the workplace drowns out the language of the world which the patient brings.

The principal virtue of this book is, as one might expect, the detailed analyses of text which Mishler undertakes. The general approach is overtly interpretative rather than descriptive and, as is the case with all such kinds of qualitative study, it is by the persuasive quality of the analysis that the book stands or falls.

However, Mishler is instructive for another reason – the same reason that characterises all qualitative research. The book is clearly successful, yet it is hard to summarise. Indeed, any attempt at summary can quickly degenerate into a kind of vacuous shorthand. Starting, for example, with the summary of his work offered a couple of paragraphs ago, one might conclude 'and so you see Mishler, too, believes that patient-centredness is important' – a fatuous summary for a complex book. (Contrast the following helpful summary of a drug trial: 'and so we see that treatment with Livlonganprosper is better than treatment with Witherandie.')

Mishler's study is intelligent and elegantly written, as the brief quotations offered here demonstrate. The quality of elegance is one often associated with qualitative research. Indeed, a large number of outstanding researchers write very well – the great American anthropologist Clifford Geertz is quoted as saying 'I'm probably a closet rhetorician, though I'm coming out of the closet a bit.'[31] And from this to the self-consciously literary style of such texts as one finds perhaps particularly in some of the early work of Glaser and Strauss[32] or the travel writing of a great social commentator and novelist such as Naipaul[33] is a short journey – in terms of approach, if not entirely of literary style. That is to say, the whole point of non-quantitative methodologies is that they cannot really be summarised – we are, where communication is concerned, as far away as we can get from easy push-button links between cause and effect, or from the world of the 'take-home message.'

For centuries there has been a debate in broadly literary circles, but not only there, about the relationship between language and thought. One view, normally thought of as neoclassical, is that language is in essence a means of presenting ideas. There are two famous expressions which have come to represent this view. One is Alexander Pope's phrase from 1711:[34]

> True Wit is Nature to Advantage drest,
> What oft was Thought, but ne'er so well Exprest.

The other is Dr Johnson's remark[35] that 'Language is the dress of thought', from 1781. (Inevitably the position is a little more complex than this. Pope was arguing, in essence, in favour of plainness in language, and Johnson was arguing that the language given to characters in literature should be appropriate to their station.)

The scientist's view, of course, is that language is there to describe experimental work as dispassionately as possible. The scientific writer is the scientist with a pen rather than a test tube, the cool observer of the way the world works, an individual to whom rhetoric is anathema. This of course is not true. The scientist has an agenda beyond publishing the truth, and there is in any case a very considerable difference between the calm retrospective of the published paper and the hurly-burly of the world of the experiment (see, for example, *Opening Pandora's Box*,[36] which looks behind the scenes at laboratory life). Wordsworth famously described poetry as 'emotion recollected in tranquillity'[37] – and the same might be said of the scientific paper.

Nevertheless, the view that language is the dress of thought is in essence the view of the quantitative researcher. The other view is that language and thought are, in some sense, the same thing. These days, we think of literary genres as exemplifying the way that the two are bound up together. We do not argue, presumably, that 'To be or not to be, that is the question' means the same as 'I am contemplating suicide', except in some very trivial way. Equally, some approaches to qualitative research, as we have seen, are also essentially persuasive rather than descriptive, profoundly felt rather than dispassionately expressed, their authors willing to wear their hearts on their sleeves.

The most elegant expression of this view is that of Vygotsky.[38] This is towards the end of that classic of mid-twentieth-century thought which I mentioned earlier, and Vygotsky's theme here, interestingly, leads him into a long discussion of acting, and the relationship between the words that the text consists of, and the 'inner speech' which the actors bring to the audience. It is, in one very obvious sense, the case for role play as an educational methodology.

> The relationship between thought and word is a living process; thought is born through words. A word devoid of thought is a dead thing, and a thought unembodied in words remains a shadow.

The final words of the book are:

> Thought and language, which reflect reality in a way different from that of perception, are the key to the nature of human consciousness. Words play a central part not only in the development of thought but in the historical growth of consciousness as a whole. A word is a microcosm of human consciousness.

These quotations are so haunting that I shall end the chapter with them.

References

1 Lamarck JB (Eliot H, trans.). *Zoological Philosophy.* London: Macmillan; 1914.
2 Mead N, Bower P. Patient-centredness: a conceptual framework and review of the empirical literature. *Soc Sci Med.* 2000; **51:** 1087–110.
3 Hobbes T. *Leviathan.* Oxford: Oxford Paperbacks; 1998 (first published 1651); www.gutenberg.org/etext/3207 (accessed 12 March 2007).
4 Virtual Experiences Research Group; www.cise.ufl.edu/research/vegroup/VOSCE (accessed 3 April 2007).
5 Pinker S. *The Blank Slate.* New York: Penguin; 2002.
6 Owen JL. A retrospective on behavioural approaches to human language – and some promising new developments; www.acjournal.org/holdings/vol5/iss3/index.htm (accessed 12 March 2007).
7 Watson JB. Psychology as the behaviorist views it. *Psychol Rev.* 1913; **20:** 158–77; http://psychclassics.yorku.ca/Watson/views.htm (accessed 2 April 2007).
8 Locke J (Woolhouse RS, editor). *An Essay Concerning Human Understanding.* Harmondsworth: Penguin; 1998 (first published 1690).
9 Locke J (Grant RW, Tarcov N, editors). *Some Thoughts Concerning Education and the Conduct of the Understanding.* Indianapolis, IN: Hackett Publishing Co., Inc; 1996 (first published 1693).
10 Ayer AJ. *Logical Positivism.* Glencoe, IL: Free Press; 1959.
11 Pavlov IP. *Conditioned Reflexes: an investigation of the physiological activity of the cerebral cortex.* Anrep GV, trans. London: Oxford University Press; 1927. http://psychclassics.yorku.ca/Pavlov/lecture2.htm (accessed 12 March 2007).
12 Moulton WG. Linguistics and language teaching in the United States 1940–1960. In: Mohrmann C, Sommerfelt A, Whatmough J, editors. *Trends in European and American Linguistics 1930–1960.* Antwerp: Spectrum; 1961.
13 Dingman R. Language at war: US marine corps Japanese language officers in the Pacific War. *J Military History.* 2004; **68:** 853–83.
14 Smith PD. *A Comparison of the Cognitive and Audiolingual Approaches to Foreign Language Instruction: the Pennsylvania Project.* Philadelphia, PA: Center for Curriculum Development; 1970.
15 Skinner BF. *Verbal Behavior.* New York: Appleton-Century-Crofts; 1957.

16 Chomsky N. A review of BF Skinner's *Verbal Behavior. Language.* 1959; **35**: 26–58. (Reprinted, with Preface, in Jakobovits LA, Miron MS, editors. *Readings in the Psychology of Language.* New York: Prentice-Hall Inc.; 1967. pp. 142–3.)

17 Bandler R, Grinder J. *Frogs Into Princes: neuro-linguistic programming.* Moab, UT: Real People Press; 1979.

18 Hoey M. Persuasive rhetoric in linguistics: a stylistic study of some features of the language of Noam Chomsky. In: Hunston S, Thompson G, editors. *Evaluation in Text: authorial stance and the construction of discourse.* Oxford: Oxford University Press; 2000.

19 Levine RD, Postal PM. A corrupted linguistics. In: Collier P, Horowitz D, editors. *The Anti-Chomsky Reader.* New York: Encounter Books; 2004.

20 Botha RP. *Challenging Chomsky: the generative garden game.* Oxford: Blackwell; 1989.

21 Gliedman J. Interview with Noam Chomsky. *Omni* 1983; **6**: 112–18.

22 Ryle G. *The Concept of Mind.* Chicago, IL: University of Chicago Press; 1984 (first published 1949).

23 Byrne P, Long B. *Doctors Talking to Patients.* London: HMSO; 1976.

24 Balint E, Courtenay M, Elder A *et al. The Doctor, the Patient and the Group: Balint revisited.* London: Routledge; 1993.

25 Working Party of the Royal College of General Practitioners. *The Triaxial Model of the Consultation.* London: Royal College of General Practitioners; 1972.

26 Mishler E. *The Discourse of Medicine: dialectics of medical interviews.* Norwood, NJ: Ablex; 1984.

27 Silverman D, Torode B. *The Material World: some theories of language and its limits.* Boston, MA: Routledge and Kegan Paul; 1980.

28 Schutz A. The problem of social reality. In: Natanson M, editor. *Collected Papers. Volume 1.* The Hague: Martinus Nijhoff; 1962.

29 Noordhof PJP. Scientism. In: Honderich T, editor. *The Oxford Companion to Philosophy* (2e). Oxford: Oxford University Press; 2005.

30 Habermas J (Viertel J, trans.). *Theory and Practice.* Boston, MA: Beacon; 1973.

31 Olson GA. The social scientist as author: Clifford Geertz on ethnography and social construction. *J Adv Composition.* 1991; **11**: 245–68; www.jacweb.org/Archived_volumes/Text_articles/V11_I2_OlsonGeertz.htm (accessed 14 March 2007).

32 Strauss A, Glaser B. *Anguish: a case history of a dying trajectory.* Mill Valley, CA: Sociology Press; 1970.

33 Naipaul VS. *Among the Believers.* Harmondsworth: Penguin; 1982.

34 Pope A. Essay on criticism. In: Rogers P, editor. *Selected Poetry.* Oxford: Oxford University Press; 1998 (first published 1711).

35 Johnson S. Life of Abraham Cowley. In: Lonsdale R, editor. *The Lives of the Most Eminent English Poets.* Oxford: Oxford University Press; 2006 (first published 1781).

36 Gilbert G, Mulkay M. *Opening Pandora's Box: a sociological analysis of scientific discourse.* Cambridge: Cambridge University Press; 1984.

37 Wordsworth W. Preface to Lyrical Ballads. In: Brett RL, Jones AR, editors. *Lyrical Ballads: the text of the 1798 edition with the additional 1800 poems and the prefaces: Wordsworth and Coleridge.* London: Routledge; 1991.

38 Vygotsky LS. *Thought and Language.* New York: MIT Press and John Wiley & Sons; 1962.

CHAPTER 6

Remediation and referrals

This Jack, joke, poor potsherd, 'patch, matchwood, immortal
diamond
Is immortal diamond.

**(Gerard Manley Hopkins, That Nature is a Heraclitean fire,
and of the comfort of the Resurrection[1])**

Introduction

I intend in the following section to reflect on my own experiences. There is an obvious danger in this – that you will think I am trying to present myself as unusually sensitive, or clever, or innovative. But I hope you will bear with me. I would like this to be seen as part of a dialogue with myself and with you, rather than a statement of certainties or an indication of the right way to do things. Obviously I think it is, pretty much, or I would do things differently – but my certainty is less than total. Nor, I hasten to add, do I want to claim that this is a unique, or even a particularly unusual, way of proceeding. Throughout this chapter I have steered clear of any attempt at a theoretical underpinning, beyond comments on the linguistic nature of some of the difficulties. This is partly because I want to present these cases as pragmatic educational problems, managed I hope in a common-sense way, but partly also because our understanding (or at any rate my understanding) of the matrix of issues at stake here is poor.

One of the most interesting aspects of my professional life is that I deal on a very frequent basis with doctors (and less frequently, with undergraduates) who are perceived as having 'a problem' with what is usually labelled communication skills. These are referrals to our Postgraduate Workforce Deanery from concerned parties who may sometimes be saying nothing more precise than 'There's something worrying here – please advise.' Within the Deanery, as it happens, they are very well handled, and the referrals who reach us are always appropriate, in the sense that either there is a problem in our area of expertise, or a need for reassurance that there is no such problem.

Over the past five years I and my colleagues have seen nearly 200 of these individuals. They range from people with excellent skills and attitudes who have been erroneously referred, to those who cause very serious concern indeed. I would like to look at some of the typical issues that arise with regard to these referrals, as a means of highlighting a number of the issues that have run throughout this book.

The basic format of a referral – although we obviously try to individualise our intervention – is that I meet the doctor on a one-to-one basis to discover his or her view of the problem. We then fairly typically agree that there should be a half-day of training with a role player and a facilitator (so below I talk sometimes of what 'I' do and sometimes of what 'we' do). This is sometimes followed by a second, and very occasionally a third, training session, and a detailed report is produced. The whole series of meetings is treated very confidentially.

As a result of the need for confidentiality, the stories that follow should be treated as just that – fictions, deriving from experience. They are not individual doctors, nor are they composites of Doctor A with a little of Doctor B thrown in. Even this approach would, I think, undermine the guarantees given to the individuals who are referred. I offer the stories here because they certainly represent typical issues, but they are not true. However, I have tried to give them a particularity which I hope will enable the reader to reflect in more detail and see meaning in small things.

The man with the missing button

Ravi was Indian born and Indian trained. He had been in the UK for 25 years or so, sometimes in employment as a GP, usually dotting around the country doing locum work, without apparently building much of a career for himself anywhere – and sometimes he was not working. He had been advised that coming to see us was something of a last resort – a way of heading off the possibility of suspension by the General Medical Council. He stands as a good example of a man caught for life in a profession to which he was fundamentally unsuited.

He used to arrive in a battered raincoat that was too small for him, always with the same button missing and never sewn back on. On each occasion he carried a plastic carrier bag with the name of a supermarket chain on it, and in this bag would be perhaps a pen, or a notebook, or a newspaper to read on the train, or sweets, or the remains of a sandwich – he had a long journey, and this bag of small consolations for the trip was a piece of his private self that always accompanied him. His step was slow and serious, but with a slight and ponderous bounce to it. His complexion was grey and unhealthy, his jowls heavy and his look downcast. He also looked in some way unhappy – quiet and defeated, aged 50-something but never young.

I always begin the first meeting with just myself and the doctor present, and I always begin by asking why the doctor thinks we're meeting. This tends to work well. Sometimes doctors are angry about the referral, and even if they aren't, or don't want to display their anger, they need to give their own version of events before any serious training can occur. And in addition, some doctors reveal themselves at this stage as having limited ways of conceptualising issues, and look at me blankly. 'I'm here because I was told to come' they will say, and if you ask why they were told to come, the follow-up will be equally concrete: 'Because they said I had a problem.'

So it was with Ravi.

'Why are we meeting today?'

He gave me a bewildered look. 'Dr Smith sent me.'

'Yes', I said. 'I have his letter here. But tell me in your own words. Tell me why you think he decided to send you.'

The sentence was too complicated for him. 'I went to see him last week and he said to come and see you, you see, for a talk because he wants me to see and get help for my communication, I mean because he says I have problems with communication, so to improve this because of the problems.' He stopped.

'I see. Why did he think there was something wrong?' Again the grammatically complex sentence (formally 'complex' because it has two verbs) seemed not to make complete sense. 'What was the problem?'

This precipitated an even longer response. With Ravi, then and subsequently when I asked him to explain in his own words, it appeared the problem was so complex, the injustice so grotesque, the accusation so iniquitous, that no words could encompass it. So he told his story, something about one of his locum posts. There had been, one evening, a visit to a patient that was not undertaken, or undertaken too late, or too briefly, despite repeated appeals from the patient's partner ('But you can't visit everyone, you see', Ravi assured me). Did he visit? It wasn't entirely clear from what he said – I knew from the accompanying paperwork that he had not, and perhaps this was what Ravi wanted to say. It was just that he couldn't quite manage to say it.

'Sorry. So did you visit the patient?'

'Oh yes, often I know this patient and after he was in hospital you see and when he came out also I went to see him, and he was very grateful, oh he said you are very kind doctor to come and see me.'

'When was this?' He gave a date, or at any rate a year, which was prior to the incident which had caused the trouble.

'So that was before there was a problem?'

'No, never problems. Always he would say how nice to see you, doctor . . .'

And so on. At best, the intent was to sound thorough with all those multiple questions, or at least to indicate to the patient (and to me) that he was trying. But the effect on me was merely to cause confusion.

He was neither clever nor articulate, but he tried to do what we asked him to do. I found, as I often do in such cases, that his explanations were not only inarticulate – they were dull. In the end, over the course of our meetings, I realised that it was always the same. I would ask a question, and he would answer in terms I didn't really understand, until I told him to stop. If I did not ask him to stop, he would keep going and going and going, anxious about silence, his voice sometimes sinking almost to a whisper, his delivery in a monotone and occasionally a little tremulous. I struggled to pay attention, and with or without attention failed to comprehend what he was saying. He made a mockery of the concept of 'good listening skills', which – well, given the boredom and bewilderment I felt – I was trying to act out. It was clear that, as far as he was concerned, silence from the other party was a demand for words from him. However, when he was very explicitly told to end the monologue, he always did so at once, with a kind of crestfallen obedience. Similarly, he was easy to interrupt.

Finally, that first afternoon, as he rambled on, I held my hand up to get him to stop talking, and changed the subject.

'Let's think about training', I suggested. 'We'll get role players in to work with you. Most people enjoy this. They'll pretend to be patients, and you have a consultation with them, and then we can discuss what's happened.'

And so we set up a series of meetings, and he would come through to meet us (myself, usually with a clinical colleague and a role player) with that same slow, bouncy walk. It seemed to rain every time he came, and there was always the same raincoat, the same plastic carrier bag or another one, the same bedraggled air. And on each occasion we gave him practice with basic GP consultations.

He had – inevitably, given his speech style as it manifested itself in discussion – a habit of asking multiple questions. We had one straightforward presentation of depression, for instance:

'So do you waken up often early in the morning or this has only been recently, or maybe just one or two times, or how you usually sleep?'

The role player, doing depression, would be fairly taciturn, and Ravi was as ever anxiously filling the gaps.

'Over the last few weeks', the role player might say.

'And what about drinking, drinking I mean alcohol do you drink alcohol or how much do you drink maybe in the evenings?'

'A little, not much.'

'And eating, are you eating well or maybe you have gone off I mean gone off your food, not eating as usually.'

It was all like this. We would get him to restrict his questioning style to a single question, to keep everything he said brief, and to leave pauses. And each time he would obediently show some marginal improvement, and each time when he came back again with his odd walk and his battered raincoat he would have forgotten the last meeting, and once more the multiple questions would emanate from him in the same monotone, and the process would begin again.

So what were the problems?

First, Ravi's English was poor. I didn't subject it to any detailed scrutiny, but I was sure, for example, that his vocabulary was unusually small for the professional context. He made quite frequent grammatical mistakes. He had almost no cultural references and very few idioms at his command, apart from a few associated with a roughly medical context (like the phrase 'gone off your food', cited above). Also he sometimes appeared to be guessing about what I or the role player was saying, but guessing without anxiety or fuss, as if this was something he did so routinely that he no longer noticed it. Once a role player rather cleverly added membership of the TA to his brief, so that he could slip it into the conversation and see whether Ravi either knew about it, or would ask what it meant. (For those who don't know, the TA, or Territorial Army, is a kind of army reserve in the UK, and a fairly well-known part of British life.) Ravi gave no sign of even hearing the reference.

Secondly, and as a quite separate issue, Ravi's communication skills were extremely poor. He had no skill in asking questions, most noticeably, and his tendency to talk at enormous length meant that he had a habit of obscuring issues that had already been explained by explaining them all over again, in different words and with a slightly different meaning. Even when he was consulting he had the same tired, immobile, defeated air as at all other times, so he conveyed no sense of pleasure at seeing the patient, no sense of optimism or confidence, nor even particularly of courtesy. It was not that he was unusually anxious, and certainly not that he was rude – it was just that there seemed to be no positive message coming from him at all, ever, about anything. He could say 'What can I do for you?' with the illocutionary effect of 'I doubt if I can help', with no idea that he was doing it, with no such intention, but with an indifferent lack of authority that could drain the room of hope and light.

Thirdly, his insight into his failings was almost non-existent. Why did he come and see us? Because he had been told he had to. This view never seemed to change. Could he reflect on what we were teaching him, and use this reflection to sustain progress? Not at all. He always forgot. Did he accept that he had a problem? Well, this was the nearest to an understanding of the situation he ever came – he knew it was what we wanted to hear, so he said that he did accept it.

Fourthly, he had no ability to study. We gave him videos of himself in action to take away and look at, and gave him points to look for and reflect on. He had nothing to say about them when he came back, to the extent that we wondered whether he had access to a video, although he said that he did. We encouraged him to make notes of our meetings. That would be the day he hadn't brought a pencil, or if he had, he would have nothing to write on, or if the plastic bag magically produced both of these items, he would scribble a few notes which he would forget to take with him at the end of the meeting.

Fifthly, when I asked clinical colleagues to be present, partly because he seemed to me not to have a great deal of clinical knowledge, they were shocked at his ignorance.

Sixthly, he made us all feel sad. Behind absolutely everything that happened during our meetings, we saw a man beaten down by the world he lived in. Possibly once – or so I used to speculate – when he was young and came to the UK full of hope, possibly then things were different. I imagined him impressed with his own daring, perhaps showing off to a young wife about how there was no need to be afraid of the great adventure on which they were embarking on the other side of the world. And perhaps he discovered then that his clinical abilities were less than they ought to have been, and that his language was poor but he had no real way of developing it.

Well, who knows? Perhaps he saw no alternative but silent suffering, and concealment of his inadequacies even from himself – to protect his family, his employment prospects and his self-esteem. However, if he had squared up to things in 1980, I thought to myself, maybe it would all have been different.

The meetings came and went, but nothing changed. I drew them to a close, repeated our concerns, and we parted with polite expressions of goodwill. I had been asked to give a report, and I made it as balanced as I could.

Where then were the limits of our responsibility? This seemed to me to be the central question.

Language support, yes, certainly. But there are a number of issues here. First, Ravi spoke no English in the home, which limited his access. Secondly, his language use was essentially fossilised – this technical term means that he had learned originally what he thought would be enough, perhaps to get through his original undergraduate degree, and had stopped learning afterwards because he viewed the task of learning as done. He was therefore stuck with his mistakes and limitations unless he began to view himself differently, and took responsibility for improving. However, this would have required insight and commitment, and I saw no evidence of the first in anything he said – the long, self-exculpatory efforts to spin his predicament into a narrative of injustice were in the end off-putting and frustrating. And as for taking responsibility, this would reach so deeply into an evidently damaged man that it seemed futile, almost cruel, to try within the limited time that we had available.

The other point, of course, is that – as with that reference to the TA – Ravi was failing to hear unexpected language, or at the very least not attempting to clarify things he did not understand. Anyone who has struggled to participate in a conversation using school French will know the feeling of not really knowing what's going on, and pretending they do because it's too embarrassing to be permanently asking for clarification. In many circumstances, the attempt to go with the flow and try to chip in from time to time is good advice for the language learner. However, the clinical dangers are obvious, and the approach is therefore fundamentally unethical.

So although language is clearly a matter of 'communication', and was therefore obviously our problem, I could see no way of assisting without digging very deep into who Ravi was, and how much he wanted to develop, and without attacking the ethical basis of his practice.

And with regard to the surface communication skills themselves, they were hopelessly weak. The multiple questions were a big issue, as was the monotone delivery – a monotone sounds dull, but that isn't the only problem. A lot of meaning is conveyed by intonation pattern, so if there is too little variation, the speaker may be less comprehensible.

And yet what was the point of dealing with the surface skills – of saying 'Don't do it like that. Ask a single question, then wait for an answer?' Ravi seemed incapable of sustaining improvement, and did not really seem to grasp why we wanted him to change. Moreover, some aspects of his poor communication were to do with his generally flat affect, which may in turn have been linked to depression (although my clinical colleagues thought not), or have been part and parcel of his evident sense that life is a game you lose.

Of course, as soon as one sets aside direct discussion of language and communication, the territory – and the boundaries – become a lot less clear. At a deeper level, one wants to talk about Ravi in the context of insight, self-reflection, learning style, study skills, and so on. These are well-worn educational parameters, all of them relevant, but all of them hard for him to understand or tackle. For example, it appeared during one of our discussions that he had been offered a mentor elsewhere, as part of the support network that was being put in place for him. I knew this man slightly. He was also Indian by birth, as it happens, incisive, confident, with a slight air of casual brilliance about him. Just the kind of man, I thought to myself, to put a bit of ginger into Ravi. They were developing a Personal Development Plan (PDP) together.

'Oh, excellent', I said. 'And what is your PDP? What are you going to be looking at?'

'Respiratory system', he volunteered without interest.

'Oh', I said, searching for some enthusiasm in either myself or him. 'And what exactly about the respiratory system?' But he could give me no further information.

You will appreciate that this narrative is a confession of my own impotence, and that the imaginary Ravi is representative of the problems that my colleagues and I encounter when they are at their most serious. The fact is that we did nothing to help Ravi to become a better doctor. Clearly he should never have been in the profession in the first place (and in the event he went into retirement). He would have been happier, and his patients would have been safer, if he had been running a small business, or holding down a fairly basic office job. This would have been something he could have done adequately, and perhaps extremely well if he had started as a young man, and never developed the sense of failure that was inseparable from him. He came to us, and to others involved in trying to help, at the wrong end of his career – and his chance of happiness in life was ruined.

Nevertheless, it was cases like this that made us all think about the relationship between the outward appearance and the inner self, and how helping one might or might not help the other. In the end, we couldn't improve his communication skills because we couldn't change who he was. As far as the Hamlet question is concerned – whether you can change attitudes by changing behaviour – what I saw in Ravi was evidence that one could not, but that in his case this was because he could not reflect. Ravi seemed like a broken reed because, sadly, he was inadequate to the life-task he had set himself.

The lady from the west

Sally was a specialist registrar (SpR) in paediatrics. She had been brought up in Somerset and, particularly when she was under stress, she had a broad accent, spoken with a light, high-pitched voice. If you had heard her on the phone, you would think that she was still a teenager. In fact she was about 32 years old, small, with long brown hair which she sometimes wore in a ponytail. When I first met her she had recently become engaged, and I formed the vaguest of vague impressions, although I never touched on this, that she was for some reason less than totally convinced by her fiancé, who was an IT graduate from her home town.

She had been asked to come and see us because she had been given what is known as a 'RITA D' (Record of In-Training Assessment, Grade D). That is to say, enough concerns had been expressed about her by those involved in her training for her to be required to undertake additional, targeted training. One of the conditions imposed on her was to develop her communication skills.

So why were we meeting?

'I have problems with communication', she said. 'I take too long in clinics – I'm often running very late, finishing hours after everyone else.' This is both difficult for the team, and means that there are serious risks of not seeing patients within the time period laid down by government as a target.

'Hours?', I queried.

'Yes', she said. 'Hours.'

'Anything else?'

She hesitated. 'I have a lot of difficulty studying. I don't seem to get much done, or at any rate nothing goes into my head.' She giggled slightly, and looked down at the table. I noticed she was sitting on her hands.

Was there anything else? Again she hesitated. 'I don't seem to have much confidence.'

The first point, about over-running in clinic, was in the documentation I had been sent. The others points she raised were not.

'Why do you take so long in clinic, do you think?'

'Oh, it's because – I don't know – I'm usually sure I know what I'm doing.' She stopped and looked over my shoulder, thinking carefully. 'At least, I know as much as any other SpR, but I have this habit of getting anxious, and I'm just about to let the patient go, and I think, what if I've missed something, or I think "I haven't explained that properly", and it's upsetting . . .'

This was the first afternoon, so it was just Sally and myself. It was fairly late in the day, and the light was beginning to fade. I was straining to hear her, she was half in darkness, and she seemed extremely vulnerable.

'Sometimes they're actually halfway out of the door and I think – no, don't go – what if? – and I call them back.'

'Then what happens?'

'Well, I might begin to go into more and more remote possibilities, or rarer and rarer side-effects, or whatever, and tell them they need to come back if they have any sign of them.' She paused. 'Actually, it's stupid. All it does is confuse them, or undermine their confidence, I know. Or make them afraid even. But I always end up doing it.'

'What have you done to try and stop yourself?'

Well, it appeared she had done a number of things – she had studied harder and harder (more and more grimly, it appeared, listening to her) to boost her confidence. She had castigated herself afterwards and made promises to herself to change. She had considered leaving the profession. However, the upshot was that she had done nothing effective.

All the same, the insight was impressive.

'Suppose I was to ask your mum for three words to describe you – exactly three, not four or two – what would she say?'

She thought for a very long time about this one. 'Caring', she suggested. There was another long silence, and then she laughed suddenly. 'Sally wouldn't say boo to a goose, that's what she used to say about me.'

'Too many words', I said.

'Oh yes. "Shy" then. And "uncertain."'

'OK. Do you care about your patients?'

Suddenly her eyes filled with tears. 'Very much. Probably too much', she said. And we both fell silent for a few minutes, letting this sink in.

'Can I change the subject for a moment and ask about your clinical competence? There's nothing in the documentation to suggest that you actually have any problems in this area.'

'No, I don't really. I'm not top of the class, you know, but I was always fine at medical school, and I'm OK now.'

'Do you study hard?'

'Yes.'

'OK. Can you describe what you do, in detail?'

So she told me. It appeared that when she went home she usually cooked something for herself – it seemed that her fiancé didn't live with her – and then she started studying, although she was often tired. Studying meant sitting in the sitting-room, at the computer desk she had set up, reading textbooks and articles. However, her mind wandered, and she often found that the seat – a hard kitchen chair – was uncomfortable, so she sat on the sofa instead.

'But sometimes I fall asleep.'

'What else? Do you listen to music while you're working? Is the radio on in the background, anything like that?'

No, nothing like that. Severity, that was the note. Severe application. Except that her mind wandered and she sometimes fell asleep. Did she make notes of what she was reading? Yes, sort of.

So then I said to her 'Your mum would describe you as shy. Is that fair?'

'I suppose so. I've never been someone to push myself forward. It's the same now – I don't particularly hang around with the others after work. A lot of them go to the pub or whatever, but I prefer just to come home.'

'And shyness and lack of confidence – are they the same thing?'

'No. Well – maybe yes, in my case. I don't think so though.' When she was thinking something through she had a habit of sitting on her hands, rocking slightly from side to side, and frowning visibly.

'So where does the lack of confidence stem from?'

She told a story about a consultant, the previous year in a previous post, who had hectored her and generally become impatient with her. 'I ended up sort of tongue-tied with him.' Her Somerset accent was very strong when she was telling me this. She felt that it stemmed from that time, and that her already rather fragile self-esteem had taken rather a battering. Then, also last year, her younger brother – only just out of the paediatric age group himself – had apparently been quite ill. He had recovered well, but his illness had left Sally badly shaken. Had his medical care been good? Yes, it was excellent, she said. She had felt at the time how much she admired the consultant. 'He was patient and kind. We all liked him.' Could she think of him as a role model? No, she thought. His age, gender, seniority, level of competence . . . Her voice petered out.

'So do you think the lack of confidence is transient?'

She thought it was. I was less certain, but did not pursue the subject.

So, then, the problem as it seemed to me was to develop her study skills, develop her confidence, and help her to consult more quickly.

As far as the confidence went, it was clear enough, I felt, that if we could demonstrate to her that she was competent in relevant areas (that she could do successful communication), if we could help her to present herself as a confident person, and if we could show her that she had a lot going for herself as a human being, that would make a huge difference.

As far as the study skills were concerned, it was equally clear that I could make obvious suggestions – get rid of both the hard kitchen chair and the sofa, for instance – that would help. There were other fairly standard suggestions that I could make – for instance, about studying actively rather than passively, of challenging what one reads as one goes along, of summarising papers, comparing one with another, all that kind of thing. And there was also the relevant question of exploring the purpose for which she was studying, which when I met her seemed to be for personal reassurance – almost the alleviation of a sense of guilty inadequacy, and this too touched upon self-confidence and self-awareness.

Then, finally, and most neatly from my point of view, there were the communication skills, where there were clearly two levels at stake. First there was the surface level, which would help Sally to use language to bring discussions to a close, and to monitor in a more articulate way what she was doing as she went along. Secondly, there was the business of helping her not to be so anxious, so that she didn't want to prolong consultations in the first place.

It seemed to me – and I hope I have been able to convey this – that this was someone who had embarked on the right career – that she was a person who ought to be a doctor, and had every chance of finding personal satisfaction in her career, and of working successfully in the service of her patients. If, that is, we could just help her to project her real self better – if we could help her to *present* herself as she *was*.

Projecting oneself confidently – projecting oneself as a leader in what is perhaps still a rather traditional neck of the woods – is I suspect more likely to be a problem for small, young, female doctors than for others. In Sally's case, it was easy to make a surface difference through very minor changes. Asking her not to sit on her hands during meetings is a good example – trivial, slightly silly, but resulting in instant improvement. Asking her to try to deepen her voice a little when she spoke – as Margaret Thatcher learned to do – is another, and so on.

(A career in education very occasionally gives one the opportunity to claim simple, unequivocal success. Here is one of my successes:

> Doctor, in huge booming voice: I'm told I frighten patients. Why is that, do you think?
>
> Me: You talk too loudly.
>
> Doctor: Really? What should I do?
>
> Me: Talk more quietly.
>
> Doctor: WOW!
>
> Me: Not so loud.
>
> Doctor: Sorry. Wow!

Yet of course confidence is not a matter of waving one's hands around rather than sitting on them. Studying well is not a matter of sitting on the right chair. Not being over-anxious about patients is not a matter of learning to say, 'Well, I think that's everything for today . . .' to close a consultation.

With Sally, in fact, it was obvious that we could not attempt to teach her pure communication skills ('Well, I think that's all . . .') in isolation. To make the attempt – to say with a purist's attempt at demarcation – that 'confidence' or 'anxiety' was someone else's remit would not have seemed unhelpful so much as downright bizarre. Therefore we did the following:

1 We talked directly to her about confidence, we elicited her thoughts, and asked her to concentrate on the (many) positive comments she had received, some of them in writing, from patients and colleagues.

2 We asked her to alter the physical setting in which she studied, and we offered her advice on active study techniques.

3 We invited her to alter her body language and voice quality, we offered her feedback on her attempts to do so, and we invited her to consider other aspects of her presentation – for example, her ponytail made her look younger than she was, and less experienced.

4 We brought in a role player to give her practice in the language of closing consultations, we offered appropriate positive feedback on most aspects of her (very competent) consulting style, and on her developing closure skills, and we invited her to reflect about how it felt to let patients go.

Sally – and doctors like her – are very likely to succeed in training. There probably is no single quality that makes the difference, but the most relevant is insight. People learn to align their surface and depth, their being and seeming, insofar as they have insight into themselves.

The man with the wild grin

I was due to meet Peter Walker at 1pm. Around noon I was hovering outside the little shop downstairs from my office, looking for a sandwich. A man passed the window, walking quickly downhill towards the building where I was due to meet Dr Walker. 'That's him', I said to myself, without thinking about it.

And of course it was. Peter was a GP, who had hit problems following a patient complaint about which I had heard only a little.

He would be, I imagined, about 45 years old, very tall and very wiry, with grey slightly unkempt hair, a corduroy jacket and shoes that had been cleaned in a fit of abstraction. When he walked, one of his arms swung out at his side almost horizontally, and he had an anxious grin on his face, although he wasn't talking to anyone.

Why did I realise that the man hurrying past was him? I don't know, except that the little bits and pieces of marginally eccentric behaviour I'm describing here are how he was, and small eccentricities are typical. And the fact that he was an hour early for his meeting? Many referred doctors are late, but haphazard time-keeping in general is one of the things to look for, I suspect.

And although he had arrived so early, I was first to reach the room he had been asked to come to. 'Sorry', he said – these were his first words – 'I spilled my coffee.' And he stood awkwardly in the doorway, with the hectic smile on his face which I was to get to know well, and hopping a little from foot to foot. He held out his hand for me to shake, but he had wrapped a handkerchief round it. 'Got my hand wet', he offered – so I shook his hand.

'Dr Walker?' I said.

'Is me', and he smiled again, standing close and towering over me. And so we started.

'Tell me why you think we're meeting today', I said.

So he began on the patient complaint. He had gone on a visit to a patient's house one night, arriving an hour later than he had promised ('which was *not* my fault'), so the family – 'naturally', he said – were anxious by the time he walked in. 'They were restless', he said, which was a curious choice of words. The patient was a man in his late sixties who had been suffering from cancer for some time, and had that evening taken a turn for the worse.

'So I tried to reassure them. They were obviously distressed, and I think the wife was wondering if this was going to be it – I mean, the family knew he was on his last legs . . .' He glanced at me a little shyly, to see if I would collude with his tone of slightly joking, slightly cynical indifference. When he spoke he was slightly frenetic, his arm gestures were expansive, his voice was loud, and his intonational range was considerable (by which I mean that there was a wide range between the highest pitch of his voice and the lowest).

'In the end I told them not to worry, and that nothing was going to happen tonight. I tried to be light-hearted, and it looks as if they took it the wrong way. Well, I know they took it the wrong way, because they complained.' And he sketched a grin for me again.

Then he tried again. 'It's a bit hit and miss, really, with patients, isn't it? You can't get it right all the time.'

'What did you say that upset them?'

'Oh, it was really just a question of trying to put them at their ease, and of helping them to feel better . . .'

'OK. But do you remember the actual words you used?'

'Well, I said that if they were worried they should call me again. I said I'd know where to find him, because after all he wasn't going anywhere, was he?'

After this there was a long pause. 'When they complained, I thought well, it's true, I can see how they took it the wrong way. But you know, I was just lightening the atmosphere, that's all.'

I couldn't imagine him saying that and getting away with it. Was the intent really to offer a joke, or was there also something of a desire to assert his power, the fact that he was free – that he regarded himself as free – to behave eccentrically? Did he want to indicate that he was above convention, to demonstrate deliberate oddness in order to conceal accidental oddness? I had no idea. However, the fact that the perception was that an insult had been offered – well, that was pretty much inevitable. Not because the words were appalling, nor even that the sentiment behind them was callous. On the contrary, I can think of doctors who could have said exactly this in a way that would have raised a laugh of relief, of partnership. However, it was too easy to see Peter standing there, extremely tall and shifting from one foot to the other, standing too close to the distressed wife, anxiety beaming out of his smile, and making himself distrusted.

I asked him about himself. He was from an army background, it appeared, and had spent his childhood in various overseas postings. His brother was an officer in the regiment that his father had been in. He had always had different ambitions. 'I used to love the piano', he said. '1930s dance tunes. Sounds odd, doesn't it?' Then he broke off, and started again. 'I was always a disappointment, ignoring the army heritage. I had to become a doctor to get back into everyone's good books.' He laughed.

'Do you enjoy being a doctor?'

He looked surprised, then blushed slightly. 'Oh yes.' I had the odd feeling that he had never asked himself this question. 'But also it's difficult to please people.'

Who did he mean? This was less clear. Perhaps his father again, perhaps his patients. He hinted at one stage that he and his wife had almost separated: 'The thing is I was getting on her nerves. I'm not good at settling down to things.' This was obvious, as he shuffled backwards and forwards in his seat in front of me. He had leather patches on the elbows of his jacket, like an abstracted middle-aged don of the 1950s, heavy on his clothes because his nervous energy kept him on the move.

So we agreed to meet again, with a role player, and in due course we did.

We tried role play with him breaking bad news. He was, as a GP, to tell a patient that she had breast cancer, that there was no doubt of this, that the diagnosis was certain, and despite the reassuring noises the patient had heard at the hospital, and despite the fact she wasn't expecting this kind of devastating diagnosis, that this really was how things were.

He did this very badly, still not quite in control of his movements, still moving his arms about too much, still full of nervous excitement, still throwing big and inappropriate smiles to all quarters of the room, his communicative competence ruined by his self-presentation. He went through the motions, used phrases like 'This must be very upsetting for you' or 'I'm sorry' or 'We're here to help you', as advised on all sides and on all communication courses. And these statements weren't credible. Who he was, his own anxieties and his hit-and-miss approach to personal interaction gave everything he said a set of metaphorical inverted commas, as if he was saying to us in parentheses, 'Look! I'm doing it right!' And as if he was saying to the patient, 'Look, I'm an English eccentric!'

After a while he stopped, having uttered many of the right words, some of them in the right order.

How did he feel about that, we asked him.

'Not too bad – I told her she had cancer, I told her we were here to help . . .'

Could he improve? Would he take a different line, given another chance?

'No, not really.'

We spoke to him, therefore, about his body language and about controlling it. And, thinking of myself in other cultures that I didn't understand, I suggested that he should learn to walk, and be typical and dull, before he tried to run and be idiosyncratic. 'Think of the piano', I said. 'You have to learn to do the boring things before you can be creative.' He nodded furiously. Did he understand the slightly unusual affect he had? Oh yes, he said. Did he perceive it as a problem? 'Well, it's how I am.' So we talked at some length about the professional self.

I arranged to meet him again, and he was better – there's no doubt about that. However, I could sense the ebullience battened down beneath the hatches, and doubted whether he could sustain the new persona for long. We agreed in the end that he would keep me updated from time to time about his progress, and that he would take up the issue of 'eccentricity' – he agreed to the word – with the mentor he was also working with. 'The question is', I said, 'do you want to put the effort into changing?' And that was how we left things.

Searching for generalisations

These narratives exemplify problems which are clearly a long way from 'communication skills' – but not a long way from 'communication.' And in fact almost none of the doctors who have been referred to us have had problems *merely* in enacting the skills set. If they have had surface problems at all, these have typically been symptomatic of something deeper.

However, the nature of that 'something deeper' is hard to pin down. The often overlapping categories into which these doctors seem to fit are themselves a mix of symptoms and their causes, of surface and depth. In this brief overview I can make no claim, sadly, to offer well-defined, exhaustive or mutually exclusive accounts, or to avoid problems of category mix. The most I can claim is that these are categories which one can work with educationally.

Communication skills problems

Easily the rarest category, then, these are doctors whose *only* difficulty is that they cannot enact the skills set.

Symptomatic communication problems

Doctors in this category cannot enact the skills set, but there is an underlying reason for this which is clear, or which becomes clear on discussion, and which the doctor – provided that they have insight – would probably agree with. The reason might be one or more of the following.

Poor English language skills

This will often get labelled a 'communication problem' rather than a 'language problem' – a phrase by which specialists might more readily distinguish it. There are three main aspects to this.

Firstly, there are problems with communicative competence. Doctors whose first language is Spanish, say, and who have been brought up and educated in Spain, have an easy understanding of other western cultures. They might very well have an excellent command of the language of the consultation, of negotiation with colleagues, and so on, in Spanish. It's just that they may not know how to mean what native English-speaking doctors mean when they say 'Oh dear' or 'Tell me more' or 'I'm just a little bit concerned about that cough of yours.' Or at a social level they may not happen to know how to make English small talk. They know all the *words* in a phrase like 'Do anything interesting at the weekend?', but are unsure when to use them.

Secondly, these problems can be considerably magnified if there are significant cultural barriers. The speaker this time is perhaps a Pakistani doctor, educated in English, who has had little exposure to western culture. This speaker's problems with 'rules of use' are much greater than those of our Spanish colleague, although their actual competence in English may be greater. Difficulties here may therefore extend to much larger areas, such as uncertainty about how formal or informal to be with colleagues or patients, and so on.

Thirdly, there are doctors whose command of the language may not *appear* to be poor, and whose problems go undiagnosed. For instance, some doctors may be so intent on monitoring their language use as they go along that they come across simply as being preoccupied with something else. They may appear distant to patients. Others may put into action a range of strategies commonly used by non-native speakers of a language, and which, as we said above, will be familiar to any reader who has tried to negotiate their way around a French- or Spanish-speaking country, for example, with school-level language skills.

The commonest of these have been known for many years as 'avoidance strategies.'[2] The speaker, in other words, uses language with which he or she is confident, and avoids areas where he or she lacks confidence. Bear in mind here just how much of the language of the clinic is routine – it is a great deal easier for a doctor to stick to routines than to pursue the consultation where it ought to go. Similarly, given the priority that is given to 'good listening skills', it is easy for a doctor to say nothing, carefully mirror the apparent emotions of the patient in their own facial gestures, and claim an empathy where actually there is only incomprehension.

Caring too much: patients

This was one of Sally's problems, as we saw. In her case it surfaced as an inability to close a consultation, but this general problem can take other forms, too. For example, there are doctors who become flustered or hectoring with patients who will not take medical advice although it is perfectly clear that the medical advice is good. Both of these categories, it will be seen, reflect doctors who have a very profound desire to help their patients. In both cases, such doctors may also have anxieties – well founded or otherwise – about whether they can cope, whether they are competent, and whether they can achieve their own demanding standards.

Caring too much: colleagues

Some doctors are perceived as bullies.

The doctor who is too pushy with their colleagues has a reputation for being arrogant and brusque – a bit of a bully, someone likely to lose their temper at the drop of a hat. Complaints here are much more likely to come from colleagues than from patients, and indeed there may be every indication that the doctor does very well with patients, that the patients admire and respect the doctor's patience with them, the way they are always taken seriously, the way the doctor always seems to have time for them, and so on. However, nurses and junior colleagues will tell a different story.

This will probably surface as a 'communication' problem because there are episodes of what appears to be 'rude' or 'abusive' language. Underneath this, however, there is again a high probability that the doctor is a deeply committed, driven individual. If you ask a doctor like this to use three words (again, 'not two, not four, but three') to describe him- or herself, it is very probable that 'passionate', or a word meaning much the same thing, will be one of the terms that is used. They have high standards, a high degree of commitment, and an unshakeable desire to support their patients as best they can. They may also have a commitment to their own advancement – that is, they may be very ambitious – but this is likely to be partly due to their often reasonable belief that patient care would be enhanced by the promotion of people as committed as they are. The bullying, in other words, happens because they care too much – or more precisely because they care in the wrong way.

Caring too little

Indifference to patient welfare, or to the welfare of colleagues, is not typically named as a problem, but certainly a lack of motivation, with a sense of disillusion or cynicism, is present from time to time. As with Ravi, some doctors bring to their meetings with us, and probably to the workplace, a sense that life is hard, that its vicissitudes are inevitable, and that the struggle is hardly worth it. This may surface in casual and careless comments to or about patients or colleagues.

Indifference to others may also be a by-product of a certain kind of obsession with oneself. In particular, some doctors have a sense of injustice (occasionally well founded) that is confirmed by the referral. More often than not, this springs from an expectation that, in effect, organisations and the individuals in them will be perfect, incredibly competent and invariably acting from the purest of motives. When they discover that the world is not like this, they become angry. And this in turn may surface in a history of arguing with all comers at work, and eventually withdrawing all goodwill. The preliminary meeting with these doctors will typically take the form of a closely argued monologue about how badly they have been treated, which is so fluently presented that it has clearly been frequently mulled over, often been rehearsed, and often been the source of conversation.

However, without the preliminary monologue there is no hope of progress. What matters is what happens afterwards. The subsequent discussion might, for example, involve a formal arrangement – a 'contract' – to leave the anger outside the room, and it will typically involve what could loosely be called a Speech Act approach. The doctor, in other words, is invited to see that language is purposive – about doing things – and the issue in communication is to reflect on how to get things done. Incidentally, it is sometimes possible – and this is a version of the Hamlet question again – to create a degree of insight in such doctors by dealing with the problem on the surface of language, forbidding them to use a few of the words of legalistic debate, such as 'if', say', or 'on the other hand', or whatever logical signals the doctor preferentially uses to lead the listener down the tortuous byways of grievance.

The mouse

Some doctors are perceived as shy.

Characteristics here are likely to include being female (like Sally, looking younger than her age, having a quiet voice, etc.), or if the doctor is male, being relatively small, and often from a culture where quiet courtesy, and a degree of self-effacement with superiors, are more likely to be considered appropriate than they are in the west.

This kind of doctor is usually referred because he or she is not shaping up, is not consultant material, has no plausibility as a team leader, and so on. The referring agent responsible for these phrases and their like will probably be a training board that is considering the doctor for promotion, or a consultant with doubts.

Teamworking

One of the reasons for doctors being perceived as 'not team players' is that they don't mix socially with their colleagues. The reasons include an inability to make small talk, for example, and the result may be a reputation for being aloof. This may be best handled as a lack of communicative competence, or it may seem more appropriate to think in terms of a generally shy or reticent personality, and to think through with the doctor the extent to which they wish to project themselves as more of an extrovert. (For some professions – hairdressers, for example – a high level of communicative competence in this area is part of the job: 'go and get your hair done' is occasionally good advice.)

A common problem in this area is cultural. For example, where the doctor who is perceived as having a problem is the only representative of their culture on a particular team, or where in particular they are, say, married with a young family at home, they may not see it as either a pleasure or part of their duty (part of promoting team building) to go to a pub after work, or indeed to go anywhere after work.

Strangeness

The majority of our referrals are people who are unremarkable – relatively friendly or not, relatively outgoing or not, but well within the spectrum of individuals about whom one says, well, it takes all sorts. Some, however – for example, Peter Walker above – are not like this. They are cases of eccentricity, certainly – but failed, inappropriate eccentricity. I went through a period of counting the number of doctors who turned up for these fairly high-stakes meetings wearing ties with cartoon characters on them, for example.

Insight

This is the single largest problem. A doctor who has insight can be helped, but a doctor who has no insight can only sometimes be helped to develop it. Ravi had no insight, and could not progress educationally. Therefore he could not learn, for example, to communicate better, and was left with his multiple questions and monotone delivery day in, day out, year in, year out.

Ravi was not intelligent, and this was part of his difficulty with insight – he had no real ability to deal with abstract concepts, or to see how they might be given flesh in his daily practice. Other doctors may be cleverer, but may not choose to develop. These doctors are defensive – perhaps they have a lifetime of presenting a version of themselves to the world (alas, the version which has got them into trouble in the first place), but they cannot contemplate change.

Conclusions

These doctors come to us as damaged spirits, as we all are from time to time. We have no power to 'rescue' them, to set them on the right personal and professional path by waving an educational wand, but if one is conscious of what Hopkins calls the 'immortal diamond' in each of us, then sometimes one can help. Or, if you prefer, there is a need for contextual understanding. Just as holistic care matters in medicine, so it matters in education.

References

1 Hopkins GM. That Nature is a Heraclitean Fire, and of the comfort of the Resurrection. In: Phillips C, editor. *Gerard Manley Hopkins. The Major Works.* Oxford: Oxford University Press; 2002 (poems first published 1918).
2 Schachter J. An error in error analysis. *Language Learn.* 1974; **24:** 205–14.

CHAPTER 7

The commissar and the connoisseur

[Hegel's] followers have as a rule taken for granted that words have definite meanings, overlooking the tendency of words to become indefinite emotions. (No one who had not witnessed the event could imagine the conviction in the tone of Professor Eucken as he pounded the table and exclaimed *Was ist Geist? Geist ist . . .*)

(TS Eliot, The perfect critic[1])

Friar: Hear me a little,
For I have only been silent so long . . .
. . . By noting of the lady.

(W Shakespeare, *Much Ado About Nothing*, IV.i.156-7, 160[2])

Introduction

If we can make any sense of such damaged people as those whom we met in the last chapter, it is because we can interpret them, and can – if we are lucky – bring to the task of offering help and advice a degree of wisdom and maturity. If we can add to this sound common sense, a grasp of how many beans make five, and a specialist expertise, then things may indeed go well. However, there are a great many 'ifs' here, and they all depend on the overarching question of how well we can interpret others in their professional role. This is what I look at first in this chapter. I then suggest that there are two basic attitudes of mind which one can bring to bear on the question, and which shift in and out of favour with each swing of the pendulum. There is the urge to atomise and the urge to be holistic, the desire to scrutinise the trees and the longing to admire the wood – we oscillate between the worlds, as I call them here, of the commissar and the connoisseur.

Performing virtue

The title *Much Ado About Nothing* is a multiple pun, as every literature undergraduate knows. There is the obvious meaning, of making a fuss out of very little. There is also a sexual pun – 'nothing', or 'noting', which seem to have been pronounced identically, has the slang sense of 'vagina.' But above all, the play is about 'noting' in the sense of noticing, and observing. Hence the above quotation. Hero, the lady in question, is accused of being sexually corrupt. She is not what she seems to be. However, the Friar, a man of judgement, knows better. He can see that the accusation is false. How can he do this? Because of his power to 'note' what people really are, despite how things may appear on the surface.

A doctor has a social role. Depending on our sociological model, we might say that he or she fulfils a certain function in society, and/or negotiates and modifies this role with particular individuals. This is familiar territory on medical sociology courses which for many years have discussed, for example, Talcott Parsons' idea of the 'sick role',[3] and all that follows from that. From our perspective, we might say that the doctor, in the role of doctor, behaves in certain ways (is sincere, empathic, honest, etc.), has certain rights and privileges (to prescribe, and to be given consent to touch, etc.) which are exercised in conformity with the expectations of society and the individual. The doctor who does not conform to these basic expectations is deemed to have 'poor professional behaviour.'

We all have many parts to play. And a person – of any kind – who does not behave in the expected manner can be seriously misunderstood. To take an example quite distant from the topic, some years ago, in a tragic and much publicised case, a British au pair, Louise Woodward, was convicted in the USA of shaking to death a baby in her charge. It was suggested at the time that one reason for her conviction might have been that her apparent lack of emotion struck an American jury as suspicious, whereas to a British audience – watching, as they were doing, on TV – it may have seemed to be simply an example of typical British reserve. Regardless of the rights and wrongs of the case, the argument ran, Louise Woodward had a problem in the States. She didn't display innocence in a culturally appropriate way.

The phrase 'professional behaviour' carries an echo of the behaviourist debate. The question that it leaves us with is whether the perceptible behaviour of the surface faithfully mirrors the professional self within. Can we be fooled? Or, to put it another way, can a doctor, or any other person in their professional role, 'perform' virtue?

The conundrum about 'displaying virtue', or about 'performing sincerity', is one that has long been discussed – and with aspects of the problem recently discussed, too, in the context of clinical communication.[4] It is a question of *presenting* yourself as you *truly are* – or, as I said of Sally in the previous chapter, of making sure that what *seems* to be is what *is*. It is also a question of central importance to professional life.

On the surface – of behaviour, or of text – are skills which we might repeat and repeat and repeat, and so learn, just as the behaviourists used to say we would. Then, we might argue, the habit of actually behaving in a particular way will make us, as it were, the 'sort of person' who does indeed typically behave like this. Our behaviour will come to affect our attitudes and to shape our personalities, and we will be able to answer the Hamlet question in the affirmative. Our habits are our selves.

Certainly the majority view in medical education is still that the surface is what matters. For example, Stern *et al.*[5] argue:

> Regrettably, there is not a single reliable and valid method available to predict the behaviours of our medical students in [the domain of professional behaviour].

They then seek to find some, and conclude that they succeed. In other words, there are behaviours which, identified at undergraduate level, will have predictive value for problems with professionalism later in the doctor's career:

> The measurement and prediction of professionalism is not so subjective that we cannot develop a means to accurately measure and detect professional behaviours when they are present.

And what were these predictive behaviours? They found two, namely 'failing to complete required course evaluations . . . and failing to report immunisation compliance.' (Incidentally, the authors also cite a study by Wright and Tanner[6] which found that 'students who failed to provide a passport photograph at the start of their paediatric module were more likely to fail the end of year examinations.')

This is an interesting approach, but once more, is this above the horizon of challenge for research? Just as the referred doctors of the last chapter were likely to wear Mickey Mouse ties, so doctors who fail to complete basic administrative tasks are likely to be unprofessional. It isn't dynamite. And it leaves us with the issue of whether we understand 'professionalism' any better. The reader will recall the extract from Plato's *Meno* mentioned in the introduction, and the way in which Socrates sought and failed to find the 'common virtue which runs through all' the list of lower-order, specific virtues.

Let us go back to the Socratic format, and intrude on an as yet undiscovered dialogue:

> Socrates: My dear friend, I understand you recently had the misfortune to fall ill.
>
> Meno: True, Socrates. I had the advantage, however, that I was looked after by an excellent doctor.
>
> Socrates: Indeed! Then no doubt, as you were recovering, you had time to consider in what this fellow's excellence consisted?
>
> Meno: I can hardly say that I did, Socrates. It seemed to me that he was excellent in every way, and I confess I did not puzzle myself with the matter further.
>
> Socrates: Perhaps we can do so now. Tell me: what qualities, in your view, ought a medical man to have? You know how I value your opinion, and the more so since this question for you is not one to be considered from a distance, but as one of which you have recent experience.
>
> Meno: Well, Socrates, such a man ought to be professional.
>
> Socrates: Indeed? And tell me, what does 'professionalism' consist of?
>
> Meno: It consists, surely, of many things, and I hardly know where to start. Firstly, he must be on time, and not late, as so many doctors are, since they have a high opinion of the value of their own time, and less so of the value of others.'
>
> Socrates: This is well said, Meno, and there are I believe many who would be of your mind. And yet, I have a small dog who tells me the time more accurately than any sundial – he tells me precisely when it is time to feed him, or time to take him for a walk. Can it be that my dog is professional?

To which Meno might well respond that what matters in this particular example is that it is the *choice* (the intention, successfully put into practice) to be on time, based on an *understanding* of why one ought to be. In other words, he might say, it isn't the behaviour but the understanding behind the behaviour which constitutes the professionalism.

In this context, in 2004 Ginsburg *et al.*[7] offered what they described as a 'cautionary tale', drawing the following conclusions from the fact that they could not easily get faculty to agree how professional or otherwise students were on video:

> We are not suggesting that behaviors are irrelevant – clearly, *what* a student does is still important. However, sophisticated evaluation of professionalism requires an additional dimension, as behaviors alone do not give us all of the information we need to make accurate judgments. Knowing how a student construes a particular professional dilemma, and what values s/he perceives as conflicting, is critical information.
>
> Furthermore, analyzing the reasoning behind students' behaviors may give us significant insights into how they make decisions when faced with professional dilemmas. Finally, these results reinforce the need for evaluations to be based on multiple observations over time, rather than on a single instance of behavior.

Professionalism is more than the sum of appropriate behaviours. Can we say the same of communication? After all, communication *is* only on the surface, and it *is* only behaviour. To say that 'he communicated imperceptibly' is to say that 'he did not communicate.'

The argument against this is that 'who we are' shines through how we behave. Our being, as with Hero, is not hidden by our seeming. There are limitations on how well doctors can pretend to qualities they do not have by performing empathy, patient-centredness and the like. This we may presume would have been the point of view of Quintilian, one of the greatest of Roman orators. Was rhetoric enough? Rather, in his view, it was character which mattered, with the ideal orator being 'a good man skilled at speaking.'[8] In this he is taking his cue from Aristotle, who makes a very similar point in the most famous and influential of all studies of the art of rhetoric:[9]

> It is not true, as some writers assume in their treatises on rhetoric, that the personal goodness revealed by the speaker contributes nothing to his power of persuasion; on the contrary, his character may almost be called the most effective means of persuasion he possesses.

In particular, says Aristotle, faced with an audience – we imagine here a large audience, rather than the audience of one or two which is typical of clinical interaction – three things must be on display, namely practical knowledge, virtue and benevolence. The speaker must know what he (and we might as well imagine a male speaker, not to be anachronistic) is talking about, he must be a fundamentally good person, and he must wish to do his audience good.

Of course the case is more complicated than this, something which is at once evidenced by the ambiguous nature of such phrases as 'on display' which I have just used. Aristotle is inevitably aware of this. The passage I have just quoted, for example, begins:

> Persuasion is achieved by the speaker's personal character when the speech is so spoken as to make us think him credible.

There is a great distance, we might wearily argue, between someone telling the truth and someone creating an effect of credibility. And much of Aristotle's *Rhetoric* is taken up with a discussion of the relationship between truth and its presentation. This in turn might remind us that no doubt if something can be learned, it can be performed. And that the art of the rhetorician (who may be a lawyer, or a politician – but may also be a doctor) is successfully to present a version of the ethical person that he or she truly is.

Seemingly truthful presentation of a self is of course the actor's art, too, and Hamlet, the most self-regarding of fictional characters, is acutely aware of the distinction between *is* and *seems*. Almost his opening exchange in the play is this, with the Queen, his mother, who suggests that he is mourning his father's death too much:

> *Queen:* Thou know'st 'tis common – all that lives must die,
> Passing through nature to eternity.
> *Hamlet:* Ay, madam, it is common.
> *Queen:* If it be,
> Why seems it so particular with thee?
> *Hamlet:* Seems, madam, Nay, it is. I know not 'seems.'

(Hamlet I.ii.72–76[10])

Below is an example of the kind of distaste that the performance of sincerity elicits in the UK, although the author rather uneasily goes out of her way to deny making the charge of 'insincerity':[11]

> Mrs Tony Blair wept last week when she visited a refugee camp in Macedonia, as well she might. Anyone would weep. But she isn't anyone. She is the Prime Minister's wife, and she was photographed.
>
> The image hit the news and the front pages, and it probably succeeded in hitting what it what it was aimed at, by the deeply cynical people who constructed it – the popular mood. At the same time, her tender-hearted anguish

was counterbalanced by virile, shirt-sleeved shots of her husband going about high-fiving and emoting, and moderating a little of his practised lip-trembling with a lot of manly resolve and righteous indignation. I am not suggesting that their emotions were insincere; what I find offensive is the way Mr Blair allowed them to be used to manipulate ours, for political purposes.

The question then is whether one – whether the doctor, I mean – should *behave* (attempt to communicate) in a sincere or in a virtuous manner as a means of being *truly* sincere, *actually* virtuous. (The question of whether 'doing virtuous things' is the same as 'being virtuous' is also a standard ethical issue.) Should he or she project sincerity knowingly, since it represents a true inner state, or should sincerity merely arise from within, with the doctor thinking about it only insofar as he or she reflects that the inner truth will inevitably and artlessly shine forth?

To which, necessarily, the answer must be – a bit of both.

The trouble with not being 'behaviourist', or at least with not dealing with 'behaviour', is that one is left with some of the most tenuous concepts around. 'Duty' and 'honour', as we have seen, but also what does a phrase like 'from within' mean? From one's attitudes? From one's personality? From one's spirit? From one's soul? From, in other words, the ghost in the machine?

I would suggest that it means that part of oneself which reflects consciously and deliberately on ethical and professional issues, and how they interact (this is the difference between the good doctor and Socrates' dog). We might as well recognise that a proper definition of professionalism is grounded in an ethical perspective, and in the terminology of ethics, for better or worse. A commitment to an ethical approach to medical education is central, after all:

> In constructing its policies, the medical school has an opportunity to fashion its actions on the same foundation that it endeavours to teach in class to its students – the foundation of ethics. The standards that bind physicians together as a profession, that distinguish medicine from business, and that enable individuals when sick to place themselves in a physician's hands constitute the ethics of medicine. If students are urged to use these ethical standards as beacons of right action, shouldn't the institution that educates them do the same?[12]

This, *inter alia*, is a little unfair on business, which has standards of ethics, too, and the introduction of the comparison here is a reminder of the degree to which 'the good doctor' in the USA is unlike 'the good doctor' in many other places in the extent to which he or she is defined by contrast, as not being driven by money.

So can one be a good professional, and yet 'perform' professionalism, as an actor performs it, without really being professional?

My own rather hesitant answer would go like this. Most medical students and doctors outgrow the communication skills syllabus very quickly, and internalise the overall structures with ease. As they learn an increasing amount of clinical content to include in their consultations, and as they develop experience in sitting face to face with a patient, there is very little that the teacher can formally teach them about 'communication skills' per se. However, very weak doctors tend to be poor at skills, but also generally speaking they are also poor attitudinally. With them, there is some purpose in teaching the skills, because it may be quicker than teaching them, in effect, to think at a more profound level, and it may result in a change of attitude.

Therefore – at least this is the conclusion I reach when I reflect on my own teaching – changes in behaviour can develop attitudinal and professional insight, and one's powers of reflection. Similarly, the vocabulary of the skills syllabus can help the doctor to become more articulate, and to gain more control over his or her education, and therefore become more self-aware.

Yet at the same time, because skills don't take you very far, because only the obvious skills can be generalised to all or most occasions, because to bang on at the same list of skills yields diminishing returns – and because too much teaching is likely to undermine already perfectly competent individuals – there must be something else. Skills are merely the gateway, and if the doctor is so poor that he or she lacks insight into the deployment of skills, it is doubtful whether there will be much improvement in attitude. Most doctors welcome the more open-ended, less precise and much more interesting discussions that centre around the role of communication, its relationship to ethics, attitude, the professionalisation of the individual, and so on. In this context, too, the question of 'doing sincerity', of seeming to be what most you are, can be discussed at an interesting level.

A good way to illustrate the issue is to consider 'listening.' 'Good listening' or 'active listening' is a skill usually advocated as important, but what does it consist of? Partly, it consists of minimal encouragers (murmured 'oh dears', and so on, designed to make the speaker continue), but it mainly consists of doing silence – of an absence of overt behaviour. One can put a behavioural gloss on to 'good listening' ('Your body language is attentive', for example, although these are subjective assessments with little scope for further deconstruction), but good listening works in covert ways.

Here is an example, from a very experienced GP (for transcription conventions, *see* Appendix). The patient is distressed about the problem of looking after her elderly mother (note that I have altered the text slightly beyond routine anonymisation, as the details in the original are very specific):

> Patient: Well my son said 'Mum I'm going down to Wales for the week if you'd like to come for a break' I can't get a holiday you see/ doctor because she won't go anywhere//
>
> Doctor: /Hmm //hmm
>
> Patient: So that I can feel I can go away/ in peace//
>
> Doctor: /Hmm //hmm
>
> Patient: Anyway my son said 'Well look come down to us' 'I'm not going anywhere I'm staying here'/ you see? I was right up to the very last minute I said 'Well if that's how you feel' I shall be all right!' I thought oh she's got her {faculties} back//
>
> Doctor: /Hmm //hmm
>
> Patient: Erm I got all the food in everything left it there a list what was for which day how to do it in the microwave, cos that was the easiest, all the other things.
>
> Doctor: Hmm.
>
> Patient: Went on the Thursday morning, on the Friday my daughter-in-law goes and the first thing she says, 'Look, she's gone away and left me all on me own and no food.'
>
> Doctor: Hmm.
>
> Patient: So my daughter-in-law said 'Knew it was wrong' you see right she got her things together and took her round to my sister's.
>
> Doctor: /Hmm //hmm hmm.
>
> Patient: So she said 'Oh all right,' but she said 'you know [name]'s not due back till tomorrow.'
>
> Doctor: Hmm.
>
> Patient: I don't know how to look after my mother.

Much of the consultation is like this. When it comes to those things from the surface of the consultation which one can easily latch on to, there is almost nothing there. With regard to words, for example – the consultation contains 2414 words in total, and the doctor utters just 477 of them. Nor is there any resolution. The possibility of putting the mother into a home seems to be in the background, but is never mentioned apart (probably) from this indirect reference at the end of the consultation, and yet the patient's sense that something worthwhile has happened seems clear:

> Patient: And I thank you very much for s[zz] giving me your time and

> Doctor: OK.

> Patient: you know/ I feel I feel at least I've got somebody that I can turn to/ you know what I mean.

> Doctor: /OK, I'll erm /oh well I can assure you at the at the correct time whenever you feel that is, you've totally got our support and we'll do what/ what we need to.

> Patient: Thank you doctor. Thank you very/ much indeed.

This is the difficult art of doing nothing perfectly.

What has made possible the successful ending of this meeting? The building of trust over the years is surely the real answer, and the patient's sense therefore that the doctor is a trustworthy man. Thus on the one hand we have the worth of the man, and on the other the technical competence of the consultation style. The success of the consultation depends upon both. Without the 'character' to back up the performance, the patient would not be reassured.

Therefore I am sometimes tired, yet find myself occasionally on such occasions face to face with someone who has a right to my attention, perhaps for a very difficult or sensitive matter. This might be a doctor, perhaps, whose skills have been called into question and who has been told – without being given the option – to come and see me or, referred by some governing body with draconian powers. As the doctor begins to tell his or her story, I discover that it is extremely familiar. I have heard similar tales of woe many times before.

And under such circumstances, what do I try to do? I keep myself alert for the false note that will indicate that my presumptions are wrong. I monitor my self-presentation, to be sure that I am giving the correct message – to be sure that I look interested, to be truthful. That is to say, I perform sincerity, professionalism and all the rest of it. I justify this by reference to my merely human status – on some occasions I am more on the ball than on others. I also justify it by saying that, buried deep below my sense of fatigue or of bored over-familiarity, I am in fact a sincere individual. What else can I do?

This is what performing professionalism means. It is a poor second best, and if it is more than a rare occurrence something is wrong. But it happens to me, and I am sure it happens to every professional person who has ever lived.

One must know how to do one's craft, as well as simply doing it. The sincere craftsman must perform. The tag, often attributed to Groucho Marx, that 'If you can fake sincerity you've got it made' is much used as a byword for cynicism – but there is a straightforward and deadly earnest sense in which the ability to fake some degree of sincerity is essential.

Naturally good communication in a professional context comes ultimately from the recognition that sincerity, professional commitment and the rest of these vague phrases matter. And even though the paradox sounds annoyingly pat, it ought not to be dismissed. Put simply, because we cannot always do our best, we must sometimes pretend to do our best.

The commissar

Whenever orders are given in units of weight, managers find it easiest to fulfil their output plan by making goods unnecessarily heavy. Thus writing paper or roofing materials become too thick, screws and bolts are manufactured in predominantly larger sizes. The Soviet humour magazine *Krokodil* once carried a cartoon, showing a nail factory which had fulfilled its output plan by producing one single nail, the size of the plant, suspended from the ceiling . . .

. . . a customer complains that his automobile tire is inadequately repaired and is told by the shop operator that a better repair job would take more time, which would prevent the shop from meeting its output quota of 13,500 tire repairs . . .

. . . One children's clothing factory, for instance, met its output expressed in thousands of rubles [sic] of merchandise by putting expensive fur collars on boys' overcoats.[13]

How do we decide whether someone really does communicate well?

There are two ways of assessing this. One I shall call the way of the commissar, and the other the way of the connoisseur. Neither is correct, and both are necessary. As fashions change, the one is admired and the other excoriated, and then the situation is reversed. And as one moves from discipline to discipline, once can see their authority wax and wane. The general picture, though, across the board, is of the steady hand of the commissar intervening to restrain the more vaporous enthusiasms of the connoisseur at one moment, while the imagination of the latter breathes life into the dull mechanics of the former at another. (This way of putting it suggests a healthy symbiosis, but there can sometimes be a mutual loathing.)

The commissar, in caricature, is a number cruncher, a jobsworth, an individual who is unable to see beyond the balance sheet, the checklist, the mechanics of measurement – all trees, no wood. The commissar is a person devoid of imagination, lacking in the basic empathy which would help him or her to understand that there were reasons why this rule should be bent, why that student should be offered a pass because their unusual style was effective, why it was not appropriate to ask this particular hospital to meet this particular target.

Enter, then, as a counterbalance, someone with the mindset and preconceptions more typical of a connoisseur of fine art, great cuisine, or any other discipline where judgement by number seems impossible. Yet such a person – a caricature again – as an individual of extraordinarily delicate sentiments, will find, when faced with something pleasing, that they somehow just know, they just feel, it is good. They are holistic judges, with nothing to say of their decisions, except that the object of their judgement is superb, or disastrous, or sublime, or miserable, or some other such value-laden term.

My argument throughout has been that the preconceptions of medical education, the tradition of scientific method, the urge for evidence-based medicine, and a societal obsession with the measurement of professional life by objective-looking criteria have pushed us towards the surface. The discipline of medical education generally, but communication in particular, is contaminated in many ways by this. We seek to objectify what ought not to be objectified, we measure the measurable with too little regard to whether it tells us what we need, we are naive about what such measurements tell us, we ignore the multivalent nature of language, and so on.

So we shall begin with the commissar.

At present, everyone has targets. This is a feature of professional life to which we are all subject. If we are teachers we have targets, if we are health professionals we have targets, and these targets are often linked to incentives and punishments, to an increase or decrease in funds, or to promotion or its absence.

And what should targets be? Well, this is the commissar's meat and drink. They should of course be 'behavioural.' They should lend themselves to empirical research design. And in the interests of transparency, of accountability, we should know beyond doubt whether we have done what we promised to do.

The most commonly expressed way of talking about targets in contemporary life is to say that they should be 'SMART' – a much-used acronym for Specific, Measurable, Achievable, Realistic/Relevant and Timely. The general approach to target setting can be used, and is very widely used, in any kind of environment where the defining of objectives is important, from setting out the goals of a large institution to the agreement of personal objectives in an appraisal situation. Thus, to take the latter example, and imagining a young clinical academic, an objective should be specific enough for us to know what it is exactly that we have set ourselves ('To get a research article published in the *New England Journal of Medicine*', not 'to get something published'). It should be measurable in the sense that we should be able to tell with certainty when we have achieved it (there it is, pages 50–54 in the current issue). It should be achievable ('One paper, working as fourth author modestly in the slipstream of the distinguished Professor Megastar, before whose pronouncements even *NEJM* trembles', rather than 'I know you haven't got a research project at the moment, but . . .'), realistic within resources (thus not 'If you work till midnight and at weekends . . .'), and timely (not 'sometime soon', but 'within the next 24 months').

This is all useful stuff, particularly as there are many people who are not in the habit of thinking in this kind of disciplined way. It helped me to think about objectives in a systematic way, certainly. Although at that time, in pre-SMART days, I was given 'TBQR' – 'Time-Banded, Quantifiable, Results' – as the way forward, but this seems to have died a death. (Google offers *Texas Bingo Quarterly Review* as a possibility, but that would be something else.)

Acronyms generally do of course have the power to mislead, and this is particularly so in the search for the memorable. It is fairly typical of a certain type of such labelling that in the quest for a summatory acronym the need for clarity has been sacrificed. Where SMART is concerned, 'Achievable' and 'Realistic' have much the same meaning unless one forces a degree of disentanglement, while 'Realistic' and 'Relevant' are completely different, and 'Timely' is on the face of it ambiguous between 'at the right moment' and 'within a given time-frame.' But there you are – acronyms need vowels, and Specific, Measurable, Realistic, Relevant, Time-Banded, say, yields the unquestionably less convenient SMRRTB.

The issue of targets in general brings us back to the usual dilemma. Is the reification of professional life possible or desirable? The question 'Can we reduce communication to a set of skills?' is, in other words, the same kind of question as 'Can we define all objectives using SMART criteria?' And similarly, by extension, 'Can governments set targets?'

One can answer all three questions against the sceptical backdrop of the Soviet Five-Year Plans which prefaced this chapter. The image of the factory with the giant nail will have a certain resonance for patients on the receiving end of a health service that is manipulating its outcomes.

The set of skills which aims to define communication differs in that it specifies a means to an end, a cause rather than an effect – 'good eye contact' is a means to promote 'better patient outcome', and so on. Objectives, on the other hand, are ends rather than means, so that the difficult middle step, the link between cause and effect, vanishes. Yet the subjectivity creeps in elsewhere.

For example, how one is perceived at work is central both to success and to the creation of the professional self. SMART objectives to do with this might include such subjective measures as 'get zero patient complaints over the next 12 months', 'be asked as a measure of others' esteem to sit on such and such a relevant committee', and so on.

And since what we are dealing with in one way or another are measures of judgement, and since this is an increasingly important topic in contemporary life, we should also add here that these questions are similar to the inevitable issues of testing theory. Can one arrive at a way of testing individual doctors which is both reliable and valid? A reliable but bad test is one which would ask doctors to spell difficult technical terms (we would all agree on how to measure success, we would have selected a dictionary beforehand to act as arbiter and guarantor of 'correctness', etc.), and a valid but bad test is one in which an examiner would follow a doctor round the ward and form a general impression of their competence, unsupported by any set of criteria. The former test is reliable but evidently pointless, and the latter one is realistic but hopelessly vague.

Commissars go for reliability, and they do so by attempting to increase the Smartness of what is measured, or by trying to make it more transparent by splitting it into greater and greater detail. Commissars will seek to improve on objectives, to make them as accurate, detailed and explicit as possible. The kind of target involved is no longer merely, as it were, 'produce 9 tons of nails', but 'produce 9 tons of nails of such and such a strength, length, width and weight, using these materials in these quantities, with no variation in quality as measured by some measure or other between any sample of nails drawn at random from the batch . . .', and so on. This in terms of communication might ultimately have its parallel in something like: 'Have a ratio of closed to open questions of x:y in setting a, of p:q in setting b, etc., varying this according to formula 1 to account for patient educational level, formula 2 for patient distress, formula 3 for the extent to which a first language is being spoken on both sides, . . . etc.' The commissar's goal is a single explanatory formula – the Commissar's formula, we might call it – which will tell us what behaviours to use on every occasion.

But evidently this refines out of existence the very thing we want to measure. Hence the connoisseur.

The connoisseur

> Beauty is truth, truth beauty – that is all
> Ye know on earth, and all ye need to know!
>
> (J Keats, Ode on a Grecian Urn[14])

Keats' rather pompous lines, I have always thought, are a sad conclusion to one of the most technically superb of all short poems. They represent the aesthete's view, the flummery of the pure connoisseur. The rhetorical atomisation of the checklist, its spurious precision, is a thoroughly unfortunate thing. It has allowed us to evade the responsibility of looking at subjectivity as it is, acknowledging it as a friend or at least as a necessary evil, according to taste. This is a proposition with which the Keatsian connoisseur would effortlessly agree.

And the question is, precisely, one of taste. The qualitative judgements that one makes about candidates in an examination, for example, may be considered without too much difficulty as aesthetic judgements. This ties in evidently with the view that medicine is an 'art' as much as it is a 'craft' or a 'science', although exactly what this might mean (again, the Socratic problem of pinning down the meaning of abstract terms) is a great deal less clear. The trouble is that as soon as the kind of aspirations which are relevant have been through the mill of education-speak, they sound much less than they are. One list of objectives, for 'the art of doctoring' (from Shapiro et al.[15]), includes as 'course objectives' such things as 'Be able to identify and assimilate compassionate, caring, empathic and respectful attitudes and behaviors modelled by positive physician and peer role-models'. And, written as they necessarily are in the contemporary language of educational outcomes, these things look a great deal duller than the course probably was, and this glum fact seems to reflect a universal truth.

The relationship between aesthetics and assessment has been explicit certainly since the early 1990s,[16] and the relevance of Hume's classic early work on aesthetics, *Of the Standard of Taste*,[17] is something I have previously discussed.[18] Hume argues that there is ('nearly') a kind of 'universality' of taste. In similar vein, Stern et al.[5] suggest that 'the professional behaviour expected of doctors has remained relatively constant for centuries.' Hume goes on:

> Thus, though the principles of taste be universal, and, nearly, if not entirely the same in all men; yet few are qualified to give judgment on any work of art, or establish their own sentiment as the standard of beauty. The organs of internal sensation are seldom so perfect as to allow the general principles their full play, and produce a feeling correspondent to those principles. They either labour under some defect, or are vitiated by some disorder; and by that means, excite a sentiment which may be pronounced erroneous. When the critic has no delicacy, he judges without any distinction, and is only affected by the grosser and more palpable qualities of the object: The finer touches pass unnoticed and disregarded. Where he is not aided by practice, his verdict is attended with confusion and hesitation. Where no comparison has been employed, the most frivolous beauties, such as rather merit the name of defects, are the object of

his admiration. Where he lies under the influence of prejudice, all his natural sentiments are perverted. Where good sense is wanting, he is not qualified to discern the beauties of design and reasoning, which are the highest and most excellent. Under some or other of these imperfections, the generality of men labour; and hence a true judge in the finer arts is observed, even during the most polished ages, to be so rare a character; *Strong sense, united to delicate sentiment, improved by practice, perfected by comparison, and cleared of all prejudice, can alone entitle critics to this valuable character; and the joint verdict of such, wherever they are to be found, is the true standard of taste and beauty.*

Hume explores the issues with great subtlety. In particular, he is very aware that individual taste may indeed differ – for instance, he specifically mentions that our tastes change as we grow older. And he clearly recognises that 'we are more pleased, in the course of our reading, with pictures and characters that resemble objects which are found in our own age or country, than with those which describe a different set of customs.' There is, in other words, variety through time and space. (Hume being Hume, his thoughts have invited very considerable further commentary. The points I make here are basic.)

The simplest point of all is that list of characteristics which I have highlighted in italics in the above extract. Substitute the word 'examiner' for the word 'critic', and you have as good a description of the perfect assessor as you could hope for.

The analogy is good, but it is inexact in an obvious way. The object of our attention is not 'beauty' (the 'beauty' of a doctor's professional approach, or communication skills, or whatever), which is a central concept in most approaches to aesthetic judgement, unless we stretch the meaning of beauty very far indeed. Nor are we really concerned with emotional impact in quite the same way, although the ability to inspire a range of psychological responses, such as trust, reassurance, confidence, and even perhaps personal affection, might be part of the armoury of the good doctor and the good communicator.

On the other hand, most pertinently, there is the extent to which questions of aesthetic judgement (or at any rate criticism of the arts, and particularly of literature), have undergone attempts at deconstruction in the hope that laying bare the bones of a work of art will help us to understand it. However, the enterprise seems to have failed. Taking the clock apart taught no one to tell the time, and the inability of structuralism to say why *The Brothers Karamazov*[19] is a better murder story than *The Mysterious Affair at Styles*,[20] although the methodology could lay bare a great deal about how both books work, made it clear that what it was offering was the price of everything and the value of nothing. Conformity to a set of norms, even if such norms could be established, given the premium on originality in artistic endeavour, was not sufficient.

In recent years, the concept of judgement by a 'connoisseur' has been mooted, first by Eisner,[16] who spoke of the examiner-as-connoisseur as having 'the ability to make fine-grained discriminations among complex and subtle qualities', and more recently by Stern,[21] who quotes this passage and – as is almost mandatory when the term 'connoisseur' is used – introduces an analogy with wine-tasting:

> Just as the oenophile distinguishes between wines made with cabernet or merlot grapes, experienced teachers can detect and discriminate between students who are responsible and thorough and those who are not.

'Connoisseur' is a word with unfortunately rather precious connotations, a slight suggestion of a Noel Coward figure in the background, all heavy eyelids and orotund enunciation: 'Dear boy, your communication is just too, too divine.' However, a 'connoisseur' if he or she can fulfil the criteria of which Hume speaks, is a person to be valued, certainly no pushover, and certainly a person with more to offer than exquisitely quivering sensibilities. The connoisseur will have the ability to observe with wisdom – to 'note' in the Shakespearean sense – and also the background knowledge, the understanding of context, and the knowledge of tradition, of values which have stood the test of time. Such judgements, we might even say, are the voice of the tradition itself, the verdict of the community voicing itself through a single expert.

Equally, the connoisseur (moving on from the speechless caricature offered earlier) can discuss – he or she can say not merely 'this is like Rembrandt', but 'this is like Rembrandt because . . .' This is the kind of thing one packages in training workshops as 'evidence-based feedback.' And the evidence base in communication, being as it is a little rocky, who better than a connoisseur, an individual accustomed to dealing in subjective judgements, to pick their way wisely and cautiously through the quicksands of feeling?

To all of this, if one considers it as an argument in favour of subjective judgements, one might further add the following. Most connoisseurs cannot do the thing they judge. They are not themselves great artists, or even great wine-makers. Whereas most examiners of medical students and doctors have the additional advantage that they can at least claim to have undertaken professionally many of the tasks that they set examinees.

There seems, on the face of it, every reason for a degree of confidence in this kind of approach to assessment. This is Norcini[22] on a kind of 'noting':

> Faculty observation of students' professional behaviour can be designed to have many of the characteristics of an effective assessment . . . First, it can incorporate the judgements of multiple experts as they observe an individual's natural behaviour across multiple situations in time. Second, the evaluation will be made in a realistic setting, and this is important given the context-dependent nature of medical practice. Third, this form of evaluation will include the conflicts that arise naturally in an educational setting. Finally, transparency can be assured by including and informing students of the assessment system's design, implementation, and feedback.

In the same volume, Hafferty[23] adds the need for our conceptualisation of 'professionalism' to be something other than a '"static thing" – a conceptual mass at rest.' He argues instead for professionalism to be considered as:

> . . . an *action system*, sharing some of the properties of quantum physics. Like particles that do not exist in the absence of movement, professionalism is best viewed as residing within a system of social interaction.

Wagoner[24] gives an example of 'static' teaching (or, as she puts it, teaching which is not 'meaningful'):

> . . . we occasionally receive feedback from students indicating that they couldn't relate to what they learned in ethics classes, that they simply heard the standard commentary about abortion, euthanasia, informed consent, fetal tissue, and so on. From listening to students, I have concluded (as others have before me) that, in order to be truly helpful, ethics courses must aid students in assessing and clarifying their own values.

The emphasis on context, the recognition of the need for 'multiple experts' and – note – the assumption that 'natural' behaviour is what will be observed as a result are all part of the contemporary humanistic view, as indeed is the fact that Hafferty feels able to retreat into metaphor in order to make his point.

Meeting points

And yet the problem with Hume's (idealised) wise judges is the potential for infinite regress in the (real) process of their appointment. There is a risk that the question 'Who judges wisely?' will be answered 'People who agree with other judges.' And how do we know that their judgement is wise? 'Because they in turn were appointed by wise judges.' And of course what this might mean is merely that we are back where we started, a generation or two ago, with doctors 'getting on' in their careers because they resembled existing doctors. Hence Hume's need to establish that taste is universal, and our need to establish that our own standards have universality.

This seems too great a goal. And it is for this reason that we need both commissar and connoisseur. How should they reach an accommodation?

We might imagine something like this (in the real world, things are less clear-cut, and anyway the commissar and the connoisseur are as likely as not competing principles in the mind of a single individual). The commissar atomises as much and as scrupulously as possible. In the end, a judgement is reached that he or she can go no further. The research is not there to support a greater degree of splitting. At this point the connoisseur is called in, and the two together agree to accept a degree of subjectivity. They check what they're doing by running tests on the degree of inter-rater reliability they get (that is, they check whether the subjective impressions are shared by like-minded people), and hope to reach an institutional consensus at least about what 'good communication', or whatever is under discussion, consists of.

We saw earlier how the SEGUE approach, by explicitly denying a particular link in communication skills between form and function, left the way open for a connoisseur's judgement, working within the limits of the 'framework.' A similar example for professionalism, taken from Cruess et al.,[25] is quoted below. This is one of a number of related reports from a team who understand the complexities of the topic well. Indeed this extract, taken from the abstract to a review paper,[26] sets them out as succinctly as one could wish:

> Professionalism as a subject must be taught explicitly. This requires an institu-
> tionally accepted definition which then must be learned by both students and
> faculty. This directs what will be taught, expected, and evaluated. Of equal
> importance, and more difficult to achieve, is the incorporation of the values
> and attitudes of professionalism into the tacit knowledge base of physicians in
> training and in practice. This requires learning experiences which encourage self-
> reflection on professionalism throughout the continuum of medical education.
> Because of the great influence of role models and because most physicians do not
> fully understand professionalism and the obligations required to sustain it, faculty
> development is essential to the success of any program on professionalism.

The dilemma is clear. The 'incorporation' of 'values and attitudes' into training is central, and requires, in effect, educationally sophisticated teachers.

The particular study in question was a preliminary investigation into the 'Professionalism Mini-Evaluation Exercise (P-MEX) [which] was developed using the mini-Clinical Examination Exercise (mini-CEX) format.' It is designed to be behavioural. A total of 92 participants attended a workshop and identified 142 behaviours as representative of professionalism. The authors 'subsequently distilled [these] to 24 behaviors to evaluate as many attributes as possible with the smallest number of behaviors.'

This is a list of items in the 'Doctor–patient relationship skills' section (the non-sequential numbering is in the original, and need not concern us):

> Listened actively to patient
> 1. Showed interest in patient as a person
> 2. Showed respect for patient
> 3. Recognized and met patient needs
> 4. Accepted inconvenience to meet patient needs
> 5. Ensured continuity of patient care
> 6. Advocated on behalf of a patient and/or family member
> 12. Maintained appropriate boundaries with patients/colleagues

Here it seems that 'confidence intervals [were] sufficiently narrow for many measurement purposes with as few as 8 observations.'

To some extent, this is the same door as that through which we came in. Note, firstly, that the word 'appropriate' is back with us again, and that it is – once more, familiar territory – used sometimes but not always. This is one of the difficulties, of course, of working with this kind of methodology. Generating statements by consensus makes it difficult to remain true to the contributions of the participants while maintaining the internal logic of the final instrument. Secondly, the statements themselves are extremely banal, and highly predictable. For the purposes of assessment, this is a good thing. The general air of familiarity makes the system easier to operate. However, we need to understand that these are, in effect, empty phrases for those without the experience to understand the tradition and context which underpin them – they have little meaning for students, and a lot of meaning for connoisseurs. This means that they are fit for some purposes, but not all, and also that the issue of 'institutionally accepted definition[s]' is central.

Thirdly, these are phrases conjured up by like-minded people, and they will be applied subjectively by like-minded people. And this also takes us back – much further back, perhaps a generation or so – to the same door by which we came in. It takes us back to a time when doctors might, say, select their colleagues precisely on the grounds that they were 'people like me' – and without some attempt to compile objective evidence, their judgement could not be gainsaid.

Fourthly, on the other hand there is that decision to identify 'the smallest [possible] number of behaviors.' This gets to the heart of the matter, and seems to me to be excellent practice, not merely on pragmatic grounds (it's easier for assessors to operate a small number of categories than a large number), but also on theoretical grounds. The more a concept is deconstructed, the more it is damaged. The aim of this kind of enquiry should be to preserve as completely as possible the integrity of the whole. We should always begin with the whole, begin with the richest of all possible contexts, and focus in conservatively and with reluctance. And behind this case-by-case decision we may find ourselves making in any of the four educational areas – of primary research, curriculum design, evaluation and teaching – we need to be socially aware. What are the expectations of the discourse community, and to what extent do we want to build on the consensus, and to what extent do we want to move it on? More bluntly, are we happy with the point at which fashion has placed the pendulum?

References

1 Eliot TS. The perfect critic. In: *The Sacred Wood: essays on poetry and criticism.* London: Faber and Faber; 1997 (first published 1920).

2 Shakespeare W. Much Ado About Nothing. In: Wells S, Taylor G, editors. *The Oxford Shakespeare: the complete works* (2e). Oxford: Oxford University Press; 2005.

3 Parsons T. *The Social System.* London: Routledge and Kegan Paul; 1951.

4 Hanna M, Fins JJ. Power and communication: why simulation training ought to be complemented by experiential and humanistic learning. *Acad Med.* 2006; **81:** 265–70.

5 Stern DT, Frohna AZ, Gruppen LD. The prediction of professional behaviour. *Med Educ.* 2005; **39:** 75–82.

6 Wright N, Tanner MS. Medical students' compliance with simple administrative tasks and success in final examinations: retrospective cohort study. *BMJ.* 2002; **324:** 1554–5.

7 Ginsburg S, Regehr R, Lingard L. Basing the evaluation of professionalism on observable behaviors: a cautionary tale. *Acad Med.* 2004; **79 (Suppl. 10):** S1–4.

8 Quintilian (Russell DA, editor and trans.). *The Education of the Orator (Institutio Oratoria).* Cambridge, MA: Harvard University Press; 2001 (written *c.*90BC).

9 Aristotle (Roberts WR, trans.). Rhetoric. In: Ross WD, editor. *The Works of Aristotle.* Oxford: Clarendon; 1924 (written *c.*350BC).

10 Shakespeare W. Hamlet. In: Wells S, Taylor G, editors. *The Oxford Shakespeare: the complete works* (2e). Oxford: Oxford University Press; 2005.

11 Marrin M. Blair's crying game. *Sunday Telegraph*, 9 May 1999; www.minettemarrin.com/minettemarrin/1999/05/index.html (accessed 16 March 2007).

12 Reiser SJ. The moral order of the medical school. In: Wear D, Bickel J, editors. *Educating for Professionalism: creating a culture of humanism in medical education.* Iowa City, IA: University of Iowa Press; 2000. pp. 3–10.

13 Shaffer HG. A new incentive for Soviet managers. *Russian Rev.* 1963; **42:** 410–16.

14 Keats J. Ode on a Grecian Urn. In: Barnard J, editor. *John Keats. The Complete Poems.* Harmondsworth: Penguin; 1973 (written 1819).

15 Shapiro J, Rucker L, Robitshek D. Teaching the art of doctoring: an innovative medical student elective. *Med Teacher.* 2006; **28:** 30–5.

16 Eisner E. *The Enlightened Eye: qualitative enquiry and the enhancement of educational practice.* New York: Macmillan; 1991.

17 Hume D. Of the standard of taste. In: Lenz JW, editor. *Of the Standard of Taste and Other Essays.* Indianapolis, IN: Bobbs-Merrill; 1964 (first published 1757). www. mnstate.edu/gracyk/courses/phil%20of%20art/hume%20on%20taste.htm (accessed 21 March 2007).

18 Skelton JR, Macleod JAA, Thomas CP. Teaching literature and medicine to medical students. Part II. Why literature and medicine? *Lancet.* 2000; **356:** 2001–3.

19 Dostoevsky F (McDuff D, trans.). *The Brothers Karamazov.* Harmondsworth: Penguin; 2003 (first published 1879–80).

20 Christie A. *The Mysterious Affair at Styles.* New York: Harper Collins; 2001 (first published 1920).

21 Stern D. A framework for measuring professionalism. In: Stern D, editor. *Measuring Medical Professionalism.* New York: Oxford University Press; 2006. pp. 3–14.

22 Norcini J. Faculty observations of student professional behaviour. In: Stern D, editor. *Measuring Medical Professionalism.* New York: Oxford University Press; 2006. pp. 147–58.

23 Hafferty F. Measuring professionalism: a commentary. In: Stern D, editor. *Measuring Medical Professionalism.* New York: Oxford University Press; 2006. pp. 281–306.

24 Wagoner NE. From identity purgatory to professionalism: considerations along the medical education continuum. In: Wear D, Bickel J, editors. *Educating for Professionalism: creating a culture of humanism in medical education.* Iowa City, IA: University of Iowa Press; 2000. pp. 120–33.

25 Cruess RL, McIlroy JH, Cruess S *et al.* The professionalism mini-evaluation exercise: a preliminary investigation. *Acad Med.* 2006; **81 (Suppl. 10):** S74–8.

26 Cruess RL. Teaching professionalism: theory, principles, and practices. *Clin Orthop Rel Res.* 2006; **449:** 177–85.

CHAPTER 8

Conclusion

This is a personal book. Let me emphasise two things which reflect a great deal of what I most believe education to be about.

First, above all, education gives us the power to use language to understand the world better, and to be able to shape it better. Empowering those without power sounds as if it is exclusively a political message, but it needs to be understood more widely than this. The doctor who has no language with which to reflect on his or her communication is a doctor without power, and one who runs the risk of depriving patients of power.

Secondly, 'theory of education' is not particularly an incremental discipline. I'm not sure that educational methodologies, say, are better now than they were 200 or 2,000 years ago. Newton was not a worse scientist than Einstein, but we could all agree (although the incremental progress of science itself can be overstated) that he knew less science because he lived in an earlier era. I am not at all sure, however, that there have ever been 'better teachers' than Socrates, or people who 'knew more' about teaching than he did.

The great Polish philosopher, Leszek Kolakowski, expressed this well.[1] He is talking about philosophy but, altering little more than the nature of the 'traditional worries' of which he speaks, he might be talking about education – or rather, I might be, if only I could express it so well:

> The cultural role of philosophy is not to deliver truth but to build the *spirit of truth* and this means: never to let the inquisitive energy of mind go to sleep, never to stop questioning what appears to be obvious and definitive, always to defy the seemingly intact resources of common sense, always to suspect that there might be 'another side' in what we take for granted, and never to allow us to forget that there are questions that lie beyond the legitimate horizon of science and are nonetheless crucially important to the survival of humanity as

we know it. All the most traditional worries of philosophers – how to tell good from evil, true from false, real from unreal, being from nothingness, just from unjust, necessary from contingent, myself from others, man from animal, mind from body, or how to find order in chaos, providence in absurdity, timelessness in time, laws in facts, God in the world, world in language – all of them boil down to the quest for meaning; and they presuppose that in dissecting such questions we may employ the instruments of Reason, even if the ultimate outcome is the dismissal of Reason or its defeat. Philosophers neither sow nor harvest, they only move the soil. They do not discover truth; but they are needed to keep the energy of mind alive, to confront various possibilities of answering our questions. To do that they – or at least some of them – must trust that the answers are within our reach.

I want to conclude by setting out some key principles and issues for the future in teaching and research – slogans, perhaps, rather than anything else. The teaching principles I will pick up in detail in the second book of this series, but I shall start with research.

Research

In communication, the whole is not the same as the sum of the parts

At least, not for our purposes. Language is, formally speaking, hierarchically ordered. Sounds combine to form phonemes (contrastive units of sound, like the vowel sounds in 'ship' and 'sheep'), which combine to form morphemes (roughly, words and the bits that are added to them – 'like' is one morpheme, 'liking' is two, 'disliking' is three), which combine into words, and so on.

Communication, as we use the term, is not like this. A pile of 'Oh dears' cannot be labelled 'empathy.' There is no prospect of us saying 'to be empathic you do exactly this.' This is the commissar's formula. If we ever succeeded in finding it, it would demonstrate that we live in a purely mechanistic world. We must act on the assumption that we have a ghost in the machine.

Form is not function in language

Language is multivalent. It does many things at the same time, and if you try hard enough to find a context, any form of words can mean anything. We can mean 'You're an idiot' by saying 'Oh, you still smoke.'

Locution, illocution and perlocution are different things. As far as we are concerned as teachers, we can offer students words and phrases to say, by way of example. Perhaps these will be things that have worked for us. However, we should not assess students according to whether or not they say these words and phrases. We disambiguate the language we hear by reference to its immediate context (the words surrounding it on the page or during the conversation), and our experience of the kinds of things that people say. We develop communicative competence, and we do so to differing extents. If we have little communicative competence, people think us insensitive, or unable to pick up nuances.

The atomisation of communication quickly becomes pointless

Linguists can analyse formal aspects of language with extraordinary subtlety. They can *discuss* functional aspects of language in use with equal subtlety, but they cannot analyse them with the same level of precision. And as far as we are concerned, the atomisation of communication – by which after all we mean language in use – takes us into a world of pointless detail and poorly defined entities far too quickly. The rule should be to break things into constituent parts as little as possible.

Those who study communication work in a (moderately) subjective world

All of the above is a way of saying 'live with subjectivity.' In fact we do, and the best research in the field acknowledges this. Communication is not wholly subjective, or we could not understand each other, but it is not so completely objective that we can prescribe how to do things in any detail.

The function of research in communication ought to be to develop insight

At least, it ought to be so where the purpose of research is – as is typically the case in clinical communication – to educate people to communicate better. Communication does not lend itself to push-button connections between cause and effect, and this means that data which are discovered empirically, particularly linking process and outcome, are likely to yield little by way of insight beyond a basic level.

Don't fear description

There is a place for purely descriptive research in science, and in any discipline. It is vital in the study of clinical communication, first because many of the descriptions we have are rather poor, and secondly, because descriptions are excellent for developing insight. Simply looking at a transcript or a DVD of what one has said, for example, can be of enormous educational value even without any generalisations being made. And thirdly, language, communication and society change quickly, in a way that human biology does not. For example, the 1975 study by Byrne and Long[2] is still occasionally quoted as if it was current, although one may presume that the older generation of patients recorded for it were Victorians, and some of the doctors were at medical school in the 1920s.

The threshold of challenge is unacceptably low

This is a serious problem. We ought not to accept the burden of proof when it comes to the value of communication – always assuming that we have good teaching to back up our confidence that we can make a difference. We are members of a discourse community, and it is through the community that we seek to extend and share understanding. Part of our duty is to help the community to change to meet us.

We should explore communication at its edges

It is hard to determine where communication stops – but it should not be pursued without limit. Nevertheless, there are two main areas which need to be developed. The first is the relationship between 'communication skills' in the narrow sense, and the other areas of non-clinical education and training which doctors require. I have discussed this at length. However, 'communication' in a clinical context has almost always tended to mean communication between a patient and a clinician who is working with a broadly counselling model. There is almost nothing about the semiotic role of communication, but it seems likely that what would most reassure a sick and anxious patient might be a fresh coat of paint on the ward and a nurse who occasionally says hello.

Lay-centredness is a cultural concept

The lay-centred ethos is a product of a particular type of society at a particular time. It may have absolute value, but we should be sufficiently alert to the possibility that it does not, and we cannot use it as a synonym for 'good.'

New parameters are needed

In addition, there are issues about the quality of description across a wide range of health service encounters. And although there is a proliferation of approaches to the analysis of the consultation, they are usually broadly similar in their aims – they attempt to match bits of text with particular themes. Other approaches, drawing for example from other disciplines (such as linguistics and semiotics, but not exclusively these), are likely to provide new ways of thinking.

Teaching

The skills syllabus is elementary

To say that something is educationally elementary is to sound disparaging about it, but also to draw attention to the fact that it is essential. Most medical students need, as early as possible in their career, to be given an understanding that 'how to consult/communicate' is a necessary question for them to ask – that communication is a discipline for a doctor and that it must be learned. They must in addition be given the basic tools of the trade – the skills labels – to help them to monitor and assess both their own performance and that of experienced doctors whom they observe.

Most undergraduates, given basic training and some exposure to expert practice, quickly internalise the skills syllabus, and certainly for most undergraduates it ought to require very little formal teaching time. Then the skills syllabus has ended. To persevere with it, to end up teaching senior consultants about eye contact or open questions, is to invite ridicule. One may therefore either say that senior consultants 'have no need of training in communication', which anecdote suggests is not true, or one must recognise that they need communication support – it's just that they don't need training in skills.

Other things are advanced

The communication syllabus proper starts at the point where the communication skills syllabus stops. It starts, in other words, at the moment when the student begins to think about careful, judicious, reflective deployment of skills, not about their acquisition. In much the same way, the musician's learning starts – really starts – when scales have been mastered.

The issue of appropriate deployment (of what to say when) is profound and complex, and involves both *doing* and *discussing*. A difficulty for the teacher here is that often neither they nor the students have the language resources to discuss very far, except perhaps to lead the conversation back out into safe clinical issues.

'Communication skills' is an unfortunate term for the discipline

This follows naturally from what has gone before. It is a pity – but we may be stuck with it for the time being at least – that the label 'communication skills' is routinely used as a label not merely for basic training, but also for education which ranges far wider. The simple word 'communication' would do, of course.

What can't be described can be displayed

If we have phenomena that are too complex to be described, defined, summarised, reduced or taken from their context, they can at least be shown. The dramatisation of communication events allows one to observe complexity in its natural habitat. A simulated patient has in this sense the same force as a real patient – a subtlety and a truth to life which description does not have.

This is the basic argument in favour of role play in communication.

Be inductive

The traditional medical curriculum moved, in extreme versions, from the formal presentation by an expert to an assembled class of the general truths of the condition being discussed (Stage 1), to the display in particular cases of these truths in action – 'This disease manifests itself in this way. Go and look at Mrs Smith, and you will see that this is so' (Stage 2). Contemporary medical education, in common with most education, moves in the opposite direction. It starts with particular cases and invites the student to move from the inspection of particular examples to a consideration of the general principles involved. This move from the particular to the general is formally inductive.

Medicine, as it happens, is particularly well placed to supply opportunities for inductive teaching. The nature of the medical working day is to move from case to case to case, after all, and the nature of the training and observation opportunities which present themselves are of this kind, too. Communication falls equally neatly into the category of things which are easiest to supply on an inductive basis.

This is the other basic argument in favour of role play in communication. It can be used, in fact, as a kind of problem-based learning, where the 'problem' is the patient and the presenting complaint, taken together – and where the solution to the problem may, of course, be as ambiguous and uncertain as life is, and as medicine often is.

Be holistic

Holism in patient care, holism in teaching – it's a sensible slogan.

A great deal has been written over the last few years about the use of narrative in medical research.[3,4] Patients often come with narratives, and in some specialties it is the narrative that is the main diagnostic tool, and in this sense one can see the role of the doctor in the consultation as being to facilitate it. A certain amount of the narrative tradition in medicine unfortunately deals with it either as a methodology for disambiguating, for finding the single line of truth in among the complex story, or as a preliminary to some other kind of enquiry – for example, where research is concerned, to a randomised controlled trial. The first characteristic is to reduce all narrative to the level of the whodunnit, where the overriding question is which of the suspects' stories are true. The latter assumes that disambiguation is in some sense more true than the ambiguity of the original.

These are reasonable positions in themselves, but there is a great deal to be said for not always deconstructing. In the end, the patient is who the patient is – the simulated patient in a role play is exactly the same – they are who they are, and if there is a single key to their character, then the character has been badly devised.

These themes are pursued in the second of these books.

References

1 Kolakowski L. The death of Utopia reconsidered. In: *Modernity on Endless Trial.* Chicago, IL: University of Chicago Press; 1990.
2 Byrne P, Long B. *Doctors Talking to Patients.* London: HMSO; 1976.
3 Greenhalgh T, Hurwitz B. *Narrative-Based Medicine.* London: BMJ Books; 1998.
4 Greenhalgh T, Launer J. *Narrative-Based Primary Care: a practical guide.* Oxford: Radcliffe Medical Press; 2002.

Appendix

A note on the database

For examples I have drawn from the Birmingham Database of General Practice Consultations built up between 1993 and 1995, and reported, for example, in Skelton and Hobbs.[1] In total there are 373 consultations, with 40 doctors. The database is now too elderly, I think, to be used without reservation as evidence of contemporary practice, and I have tried to draw on it only in order to illustrate points which are relatively resistant to the vagaries of time.

Transcription conventions

Most transcription conventions derive ultimately from those developed by Gail Jefferson, and applied by the sociolinguists of the 1960s. Jefferson's conventions are conveniently available in Atkinson and Heritage.[2] The conventions used here are in part adapted from these, in a very much simplified form.

It goes without saying that any transcription is imperfect, and loses a great deal of what has happened.

1 All pronunciations are regularised to standard UK English, except for a few marginal cases. *Yeah, gonna, dunno, nope* are all recognised. Brief interjections are regularised to *hmm, erm* and *uhm*.
2 Only names in the public domain appear. Otherwise, *<Fir>* appears for a first name, and *<Fam>* for a family name. Where more than one such name occurs, they are numbered *<Fir1>*, etc.
3 Where there is a clearly wrong pronunciation (e.g. of a drug name), the mistaken pronunciation is rendered thus: {*stepascope*} (for 'stethoscope'). Only letters of the Roman alphabet are used to capture pronunciations.

Where a speaker embarks on a word and abandons it, this appears in the text as, for example, '*I und[erstand] I know what you mean, doctor.*' If the abandoned word cannot be identified with certainty, it appears as, for example, '*I [zzz] I know what you mean, doctor.*'

4 Silences of 1 second or more are rendered as, for example, *<silence12>*, indicating a silence of 12 seconds. Silences of less than 1 second are ignored.

5 Certain non-language activities are recognised, for example *<laugh>*, *<cry>*, *<write>*, where the activity is of duration more than 1 second. As above, the duration is written in numerals following the descriptive term. Physical examinations are rendered as *<PhysS>* at the beginning, *<PhysF>* at the end. Categories such as *<write>* are only included if the transcriber (who has access to tape only) is certain of the activity.

6 Interruptions, or any instance of two people's speech overlapping, are recognised by an oblique at the end of the word during which the overlap begins. In the interests of readability, a series of short interjections by a second speaker, such as repeated '*hmm*'s, are placed together at the end of the first speaker's turn, thus:

> Patient: *So I've been feeling/ a bit down doctor/, really fed up.*

> Doctor: */Hmm /hmm. I'm sorry to hear it.*

References

1 Skelton JR, Hobbs FDR. Concordancing: use of language-based research in medical communication. *Lancet.* 1999; **353:** 108–11.

2 Atkinson J, Heritage J, editors. *Structures of Social Interaction: studies in conversation analysis.* London: Collins; 1987.

Index